The Personal Trainers Association
PROPTA Nutrition Tech Certification Course Study Guide

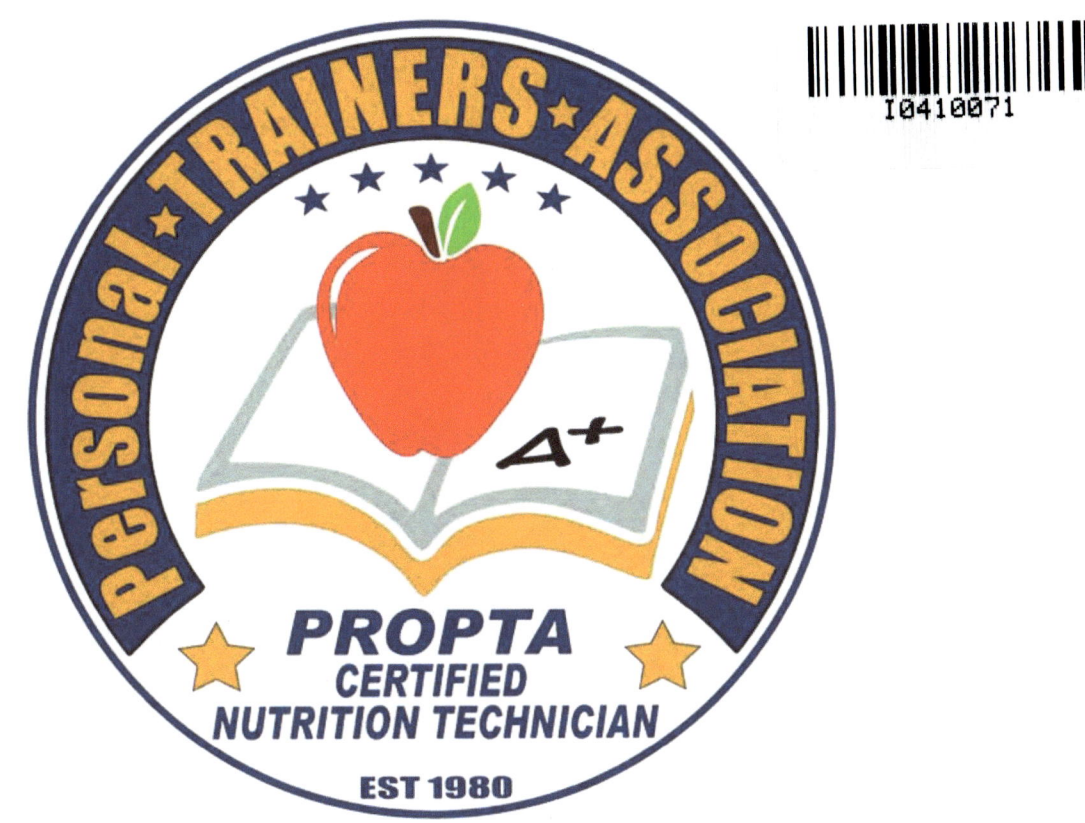

PROPTA CERTIFIED NUTRITION TECHNICIAN
EST 1980

Author

Joseph E. Antouri, CEO – CHAIRMAN -- Founder

Before engaging in any exercise or diet, you must check with your physician.

Index

Confidential activity records

Congratulations. We are pleased that you have registered for the PROPTA Nutrition Tech Certification. The format and content of PROPTA's training and certification programs are designed to provide an individualized learning experience that will contribute to your success as a Nutrition advisor. This study guide will be a useful learning and preparation tool when used in conjunction with *PROPTA Nutrition Tech Certification course manual.*

PROPTA Mission:

As the world's largest Personal Trainers and Nutrition Certification educator, PROPTA delivers comprehensive cognitive and practical education for fitness professionals, grounded in industry research, using both traditional and innovative modalities. PROPTA upholds Basic Exercise Standards and Guidelines for safe fitness practice.

PROPTA Certification written and practical examinations are accredited by Vital Research and proven experience. PROPTA is proud to announce that it has been granted approval status from the California State Approving Agency for Veteran, and approval from the Bureau Private Post Secondary and Vocational Education approval, GI Bill Approval, and also Officially Endorsed by the International Federation of Fitness and Bodybuilding League the IFBB PRO League, the largest fitness organization in the world that is recognized by the Olympic committee and many foreign Universities in many languages. PROPTA is the official certification of many foreign countries and the Official Certification for the IFBB PRO League, the Official Certification of the MMA and was recently endorsed by the Founder of the UFC Mr. Art Davie and the Official Certification Authority for the Powerhouse Gym International.

PROPTA, IFBB PRO League and other logos are trademarks or registered trademarks and are used only for informational purposes at to the owner's benefit, without intent to infringe.

PROPTA Nutrition Tech Certification Course Study Guide

WHAT TO BRING TO THE WORKSHOP

• All study materials (for certifications only)
• Registration confirmation
• Confortable clothing.
• Clipboard or notebook
• Pens, pencils, highlighters, etc.
• Photo ID
• Lunch and snacks (Meals are not provided.)

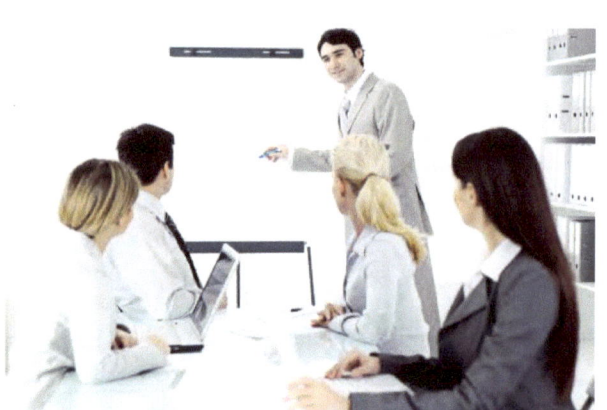

CPR certification* is required for all PROPTA certifications. If you have a current card at the time of the workshop, bring it with you. If not, send a copy to PROPTA's main office after receiving notice to do so. Test results will be sent via email to all students. Please don't call the office, we will inform you in time.

Clinical hours:

All students are required to do 20 clinical hours for this course. Clinical hours are hours for practice what you learned in the workshop to improve your teaching skills and to help you pass the practical exam.

Clinical hours must be done with a PROPTA director. Please set up time to properly execute and complete your clinical hours. Call PROPTA office for additional information at 818-766-3317

RETEST and CHALLENGE SCHEDULE

Nutrition Tech Certification course

Students may retest or challenge the course with the practical exam only. A fee of $100 US Dollars is to be paid in advance by calling the corporate office at 818-766-3317 to schedule the retest with a PROPTA director only. The written exam can be challenged along with the practical exam and must be proctored. The course fee will never be waived or discounted.

If student do not pass the challenge exams, student must take or retake the course with practical or hire a director to help correct the issue. A fee of $100 US Dollars will be charged for the retake and a fee of $100 US Dollars will be charged for hiring a director.

ARRIVAL

Please arrive 30 minutes prior to the scheduled workshop time. (If you are retesting, see above.) this will help to avoid delays, and ensure that everyone checks in before the workshop begins and completes all necessary paperwork.

WHAT TO WEAR

Be prepared for temperature changes throughout the day. Wear comfortably.

PARKING and DIRECTIONS

It is recommended that you call the host facility in advance to inquire about directions and parking information. Check your emails for such contacts or locations.

NO REFUNDS

Please refer to PROPTA's policy on cancellation; PROPTA does not refund any money to any one for any course at any time.

MEALS ARE NOT PROVIDED

Course Learning Objectives

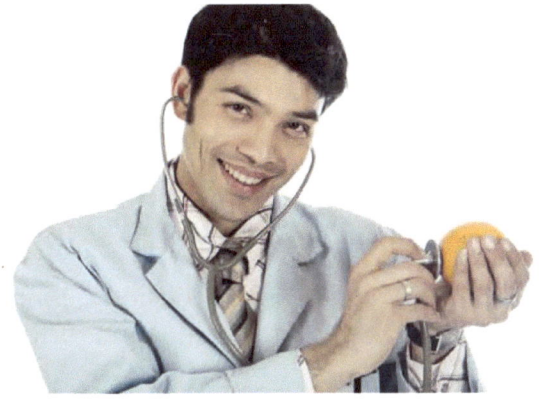

1.   Gain knowledge of essential and fundamental nutrition.

2.   Understand the prevalence of obesity and its health risks in the United States.

3.   Learn how to evaluate body weight using various methods.

4.   Recognize both safe and unsafe approaches to weight loss or Fat loss and which methods are most effective.

5.   Learn how to best maintain a new goal weight.

6.   Learn how to manage client setbacks and weight loss plateaus.

7.   Identify various guidelines on structuring an effective Fat loss program.

8.   Comprehend a client's readiness to engage in a weight loss program and what the stages of change are.

9.   Understand how to motivate clients through effective goal setting and record keeping.

10.   Understand the process of teaching.

11.   Obtain and learn the pros and cons to group vs. individual counseling.

12.   Discover the benefits of exercise and its significance to a healthy weight.

13.   Learn the essential components of an effective fitness program.

14.   Learn how to operate as a business and make money.

15.   Understand the importance of legal, professional ethical responsibilities when working in the field.

16.   Understand the importance of checking with individuals States on their guidelines and regulations dealing with weight loss and weight loss programs.

17.   Understand the importance of record keeping and essential documents in a weight loss program.

18.   Obtain useful resources in the form of web sties and many various books.

Basic Nutrition

A.   Dietary Guidelines

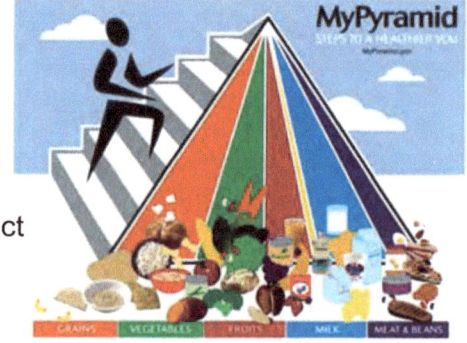

People make the wrong food choices every day at every meal. Whether these choices seem trivial or significant, they can have a major impact on health and body weight, energy and most important behavior. Proper and Healthful and balanced eating is one of the best personal investments anyone can make. Good nutrition and physical fitness activity are the factors behind good health. There is no secret to a healthy eating and a healthy lifestyle, just solid proper advice.

The My Pyramid Food Guidance System

In 2005, the USDA changed "The Food Guide Pyramid" concept to "MyPyramid Food Guidance System".   The Pyramid now has a new look with six different colored bands that represent the five food groups: grains (orange), vegetables (green), fruits (red), milk (blue), meats/beans (purple), and fats/oils (yellow).

On the new Pyramid, individual foods and numbers of servings per food group are not provided as they were on the previous version of the Food Pyramid. Instead, the key to the new graphic is to lead people to the web site www.mypyramid.gov for a more interactive experience.

The MyPyramid symbol holds several important key messages:

• **Activity:** The figure climbing the Pyramid represents the importance of daily physical activity.

• **Variety:** The six colored bands indicate eating a variety of healthy foods each day.

• **Gradual improvement:** The words "Steps to a Healthier You" suggest that health benefits can be made by taking small steps to improve your diet and lifestyle.

• **Personalization:** MyPyramid allows you to discover your own personal needs within each food group.

• **Proportionality:** Each band on the Pyramid has a different width showing the relative amounts of food a person should choose from each food group.

• **Moderation:** On the Pyramid each band also starts wide at the bottom and narrows at the top. This depicts eating foods in moderation. Foods within each group that contain little to no added fat and sugar are represented at its widest point and foods you should have less of with more sugar and fats are represented at the narrow top.

• **MyPyramid Plan:** This tool will quickly estimate calorie needs along with a food plan. Individuals can print out a mini-poster of their food plan along with a worksheet to help keep track of progress.

• **Inside the Pyramid-** This section provides in-depth information about each food group including suggested serving sizes, how much is needed and how to choose the best foods in that group.

• **Adore your Fruits:** The more variety of fruit the more nutritional punch. Eat a variety of fruits including fresh, frozen canned or dried rather than fruit juice for most fruit choices. Fruits are excellent sources of vitamins A and C as well as potassium.
In their whole form they are great sources of fiber as well.

One serving of fruit equals 1 cup of fruit or 100 percent fruit juice or ½ cup dried fruit. Based on a 2,000 calorie diet 1/2 cups of fruit is needed daily.

• **Color up Your Veggies:** The more color in your veggies, the more nutritional punch. Eat more dark green veggies, such as kale, spinach, broccoli and other dark green leafy vegetables; orange veggies such as pumpkin, carrots, and sweet potato; and go for something different with beans and peas such as lentils, kidney beans and garbanzo beans. Vegetables can be raw, cooked, fresh, frozen, canned or dried. They provide loads of vitamins, minerals, antioxidants and fiber and as an added bonus they are low in calories.

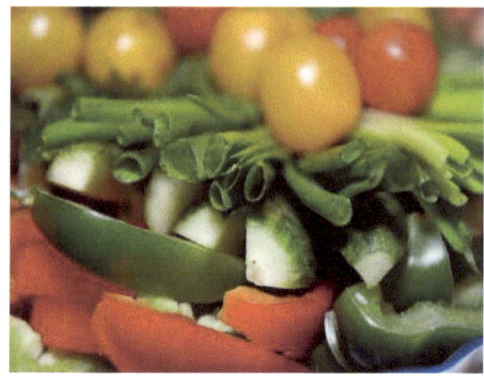

One serving of vegetables equals 1 cup raw or cooked vegetables or vegetable juice or 2 cups raw leafy greens.

Based on a 2,000 calorie diet 2.5 cups of vegetables are needed daily.

• **Chalk up one for Calcium:** This Group consists of milk, yogurt and cheese. Fat-free or low-fat foods from this group are recommended.   Dairy foods are loaded with calcium, vitamin D, potassium and protein.

One serving of the milk group is equal to 1 cup of milk or yogurt, 1.5 ounces natural cheese or 2 ounces of processed cheese.

• **Go for the Grain:** This Group is made up of wheat, rice, oats, cornmeal, barley and other cereal grains such as breads, pasta, rice, cereal, tortilla, crackers, popcorn, etc.…

Grains are an important source of complex carbohydrates and an essential source of energy. They are also an important source of fiber and other essential nutrients. The grain group is split into two groups: whole grains and refined grains.

Consume half of the grains needed daily as "whole" grains. Eat at least 3 ounces (out of the 6 ounces needed daily based on a 2,000 calorie diet) of whole-grain cereals, breads, crackers, rice (brown or wild) or pasta (whole wheat) daily. Check the ingredient list to see if the grain in the product is listed as "whole".

Portion sizes examples in the grain group include 1 slice of bread, 2 cups of popcorn, ½ cup cooked rice, ½ cup cooked pasta, ½ cup cooked cereal and 1- 6" tortilla.

• **Choose Lean Proteins:** This Group consists of meat, poultry, fish, dry beans or peas, nuts and seeds. Foods in this group provide plenty of protein. In addition, these foods are excellent sources of B vitamins, vitamin E, iron, zinc and magnesium. Choose lean or low fat foods within this group.

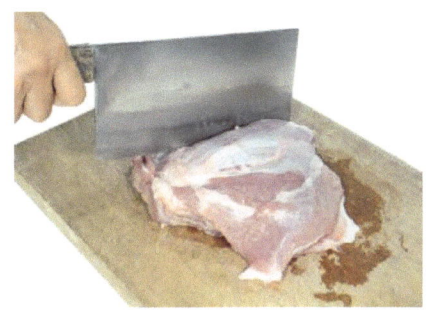

Check for key words such as "loin" or "round" to ensure a lean choice. Leave skin off of poultry and bake, broil or grill to cut down on fat in cooking. Read food labels! Vary protein choices.

• **Go Easy on the Fats:** The Oil Group consists of fats or oils that are liquid at room temperature such as olive oil, canola oil, and sunflower oil. Most of the fats that you eat should be made up of "healthy" fats: polyunsaturated (PUFA) or monounsaturated (MUFA). Oils are major sources of these types of healthier fats.

DIETARY GUIDELINE FOR AMERICANS

Why are the Dietary Guidelines important?

They form the basis of Federal nutrition policy, education, outreach, and food assistance programs used by consumers, industry, nutrition educators and health professionals. All Federal dietary guidance for the public is required to be consistent with the DGA. The guidelines provide the scientific basis for the government to speak in a consistent and uniform manner. They are used in the development of materials, messages, tools and programs to communicate healthy eating and physical activity to the public.

How do the Dietary Guidelines Advisory Committee (DGAC) Report and the Dietary Guidelines for Americans relate to each other?

The DGAC Report is a scientific advisory report and presents the recommendations of the external 2010 Dietary Guidelines Advisory Committee to the Secretaries of USDA and HHS for use in updating the official Dietary Guidelines for Americans. The DGAC Report is written for the Federal government as the basis for developing the Dietary Guidelines for Americans (DGA).

Comments from Federal agencies and the public are considered in the development of the DGA. The DGA is intended for policy makers, nutrition educators and health professionals in developing nutrition policy, nutrition education messages.

Why are the Dietary Guidelines only for ages 2 years and older?

The DGA has always focused on adults and children 2 years of age and older. Children under 2 years of age are not included because their nutritional needs and eating patterns vary by their developmental stage and differ substantially from those of older children and adults. A separate committee for reviewing nutrition and physical activity needs of pregnant women and children from birth to 2 years old could be beneficial as it would be made up of

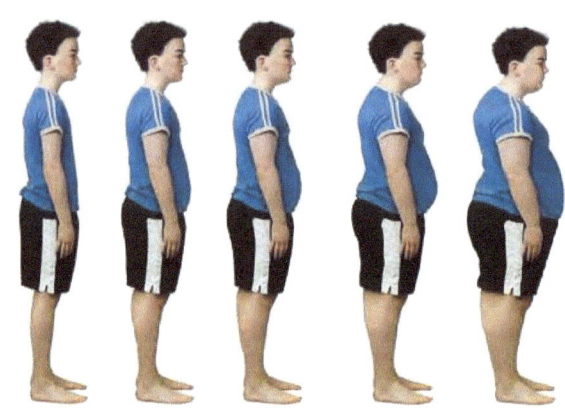

scientists and nutrition professionals who are experts in those very specialized topic areas of infant development and infant feeding practices.

Why are the Dietary Guidelines revised every five years?

This periodic review is mandated under the 1990 National Nutrition Monitoring and Related Research Act (Public Law 101-445, Section 301 [7 U.S.C. 5341], Title III). The DGA is required to be based on the preponderance of current scientific and medical knowledge and to be released by the Secretaries of USDA and HHS every five years.

Dietary "Key Recommendations" for each specific Guideline or access the website at www.healthierus.gov/dietary guidelines

ADEQUATE NUTRIENTS WITHIN CALORIE NEEDS

> • Consume a variety of nutrient-dense foods and beverages within the basic food groups that limit the intake of saturated and trans fats, cholesterol, added sugars, salt, and alcohol.

> • Meet recommended intakes within energy needs according to each individual and his activity level. Access intake may lead to obesity and health issues.

WEIGHT MANAGEMENT

• To maintain body weight in a healthy range, balance calories from foods and beverages with calories expended.

• To prevent gradual weight gain over time, make small decreases in food and beverage calories and increase physical activity.

PHYSICAL ACTIVITY

• Engage in regular physical activity every day and reduce sedentary activities to promote health, psychological well-being, and a healthy body weight. Keep in mind that body weight to every individual is different according to the calorie intake and calorie expenditure.

• To reduce the risk of chronic disease in adulthood: Engage in at least 30 minutes of moderate-intensity physical activity, above usual activity at work or home on al least 4 days of the week.

• For most people, greater health benefits can be obtained by engaging in physical activity of more vigorous intensity or longer duration.

• Achieve physical fitness by including cardiovascular conditioning, stretching exercises for flexibility, and resistance exercises , calisthenics for muscle strength and endurance. It all depend on the age and the life style of each person.

FOODGROUPS

PROTEIN

• Consume high and complete quality protein such as fish, chicken, beef, eggs, turkey each meal sufficient amount that equals to .8 gram per pound for non athletic persons, 1 gram per pound for athletic persons and 1.5 gram or above for advanced or professional athletes.

FRUITS & VEGETABLES

• Consume a sufficient amount of fruits and vegetables while staying within energy needs. Two cups of fruit and 2½ cups of vegetables per day are recommended for a 2,000-calorie intake, with higher or lower amounts depending on the calorie level and the activity level for each individual.

• Choose a variety of fruits and vegetables each day. In particular, select from all five vegetable subgroups (dark green, orange, legumes, starchy vegetables, and other vegetables) several times a week.

WHOLE GRAIN

• Consume 1 or more ounce-equivalent of whole-grain products per day, with the rest of the recommended grains coming from enriched or whole-grain products at least half the grains should come from whole grains.

FATS

• Consume less than 10 percent of calories from saturated fatty acids and less than 300 mg/day of cholesterol, and keep trans fatty acid consumption as low as possible.

• Keep total fat intake below 25 percent of calories, with most fats coming from sources of polyunsaturated and monounsaturated fatty acids, such as fish, nuts, and vegetable oils.

• When selecting and preparing meat, poultry, dry beans, and milk or milk products, make choices that are lean low-fat, or fat-free, pay attention to expiration dates.

• Limit intake of fats and oils high in saturated and/or trans fatty acids, and choose products low in such fats and oils.

Keep in mind that the body will make cholesterol if you don't consume it. So it is better that you try to control the intake than the body trying to manufacture it.

CARBOHYDRATES

• Choose fiber-rich fruits, vegetables, and whole grains often.

• Choose and prepare foods and beverages with little added sugars or caloric sweeteners, such as amounts suggested by the USDA Food Guide.

• Reduce the incidence of dental caries by practicing good oral hygiene and consuming sugar- and starch-containing foods and beverages less frequently.

SODIUM AND POTASSIUM

• Consume less than 2,300 mg (approximately 1 teaspoon of salt) of sodium per day. If you can not ad any salt to any food then the amount will be much less. Remember that all food contains sodium naturally.

• Choose and prepare foods with little or NO salt. At the same time, consume potassium- rich foods, such as fruits and vegetables.

ALCOHOLIC BEVERAGES

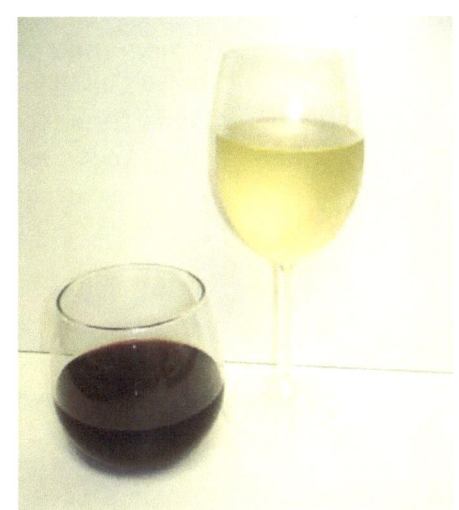

• Those who choose to drink alcoholic beverages should do so sensibly and in moderation.

• Alcoholic beverages should not be consumed by some individuals, including those who cannot restrict their alcohol intake, women of childbearing age who may become pregnant, pregnant and lactating women, children and adolescents, individuals taking medications that can interact with alcohol, and those with specific medical conditions.

• Alcoholic beverages should be avoided by individuals engaging in activities that require attention, skill, or coordination, such as driving or operating machinery.

• Drinking alcohol will shut down and cease the production on hormones in the body for over 72 hours until the liver has cleared the alcohol out of the system.

FOOD SAFETY

To avoid microbial foodborne illness:

• Use a different cutting board for each food group.

• Clean hands, food contact surfaces, and fruits and vegetables.

• Separate the raw from cooked and ready-to-eat foods while shopping, preparing, or storing them.

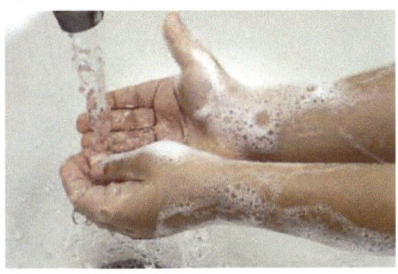

• Cook foods to a safe temperature to kill microorganisms.

• Chill (refrigerate) perishable food promptly and defrost foods properly.

• Avoid raw (unpasteurized) milk or any products made from unpasteurized milk, raw or partially cooked eggs or foods containing raw eggs, raw or undercooked meat and poultry, unpasteurized juices, and raw sprouts. Note: The Dietary Guidelines for Americans 2003 also contains additional recommendations for specific populations. The full document is available at: www.healthierus.gov/dietary guidelines

A Little More INFO on Fats:

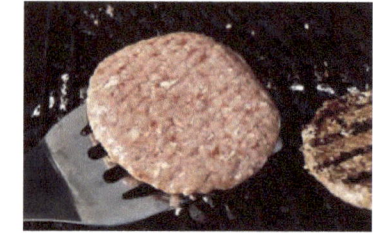

Dietary fat is an important part of a healthy diet. Fats supply energy and essential fatty acids and they help absorb the fat-soluble vitamins A, D, E and K. Fat also help in hormonal production so the body operates efficiently.

The key is choosing foods sensibly that will not provide too much fat or the wrong type of fat. Eating too much fat, no matter what type it is, will provide excess calories. There are different types of fat. The main types are saturated and unsaturated fats.

Saturated fats can increase the risk for heart disease by raising the blood cholesterol. Saturated fats are found mainly in animal food.

Unsaturated fat does not increase blood cholesterol and can even help to lower blood cholesterol levels.

There are two types of unsaturated fats "mono-unsaturated & polyunsaturated fats. Unsaturated fats are found mainly in vegetables and fish oils.

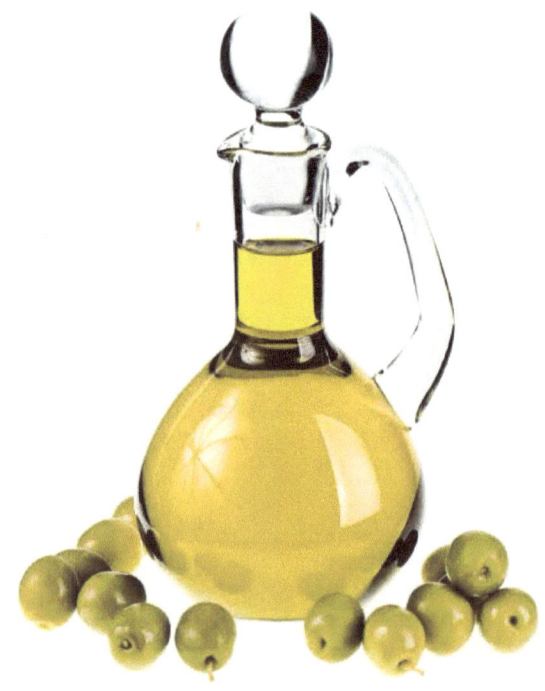

These fats are another type of fat that can significantly raise blood cholesterol levels. Trans fats are produced when unsaturated fats go through a process called partial hydrogenation.

Hydrogenation is a process that makes unsaturated fats more saturated and therefore more stable and solid at room temperature such as stick margarine. Stick margarine starts out as a vegetable oil and goes through hydrogenation by becoming more solid at room temperature.

Trans fats are also found in cookies, crackers, and other commercial baked goods made with partially hydrogenated vegetables oils as well as French fries, donuts and other commercially fried foods.

Trans fats can be just as dangerous to heart health then saturated fats. They can raise LDL (or the bad blood cholesterol) and tend to lower HDL (or the good blood cholesterol).

At the start of 2006, the FDA made it mandatory for food labels to contain the amount of trans fat in food products. Since that time, many manufacturers have opted to remove this "bad" fat from their products.

Dietary cholesterol is different than dietary fat in that it does not provide energy to the body and therefore does not have calories. Cholesterol is a fat like substance but is not fat itself.

Cholesterol has different functions than fat in the body and has a different structure than fat. Cholesterol is part of every body cell and is part of some hormones.   Cholesterol helps the body digest and absorb fat.

With the help of sunlight, cholesterol in your skin can change to Vitamin D. The body does need some cholesterol for normal function but too much cholesterol in the bloodstream has been linked to heart disease.

Cholesterol is found in most animal foods and is also produced in the body by the liver. Experts recommend no more than 300 milligrams of dietary cholesterol per day. Dietary cholesterol does not automatically become blood cholesterol.

Total fat intake, especially saturated fat, has a more significant effect on blood cholesterol levels than dietary cholesterol alone does.

The following will help to keep the diet low in saturated fat, trans fat and cholesterol and moderate in total fat:

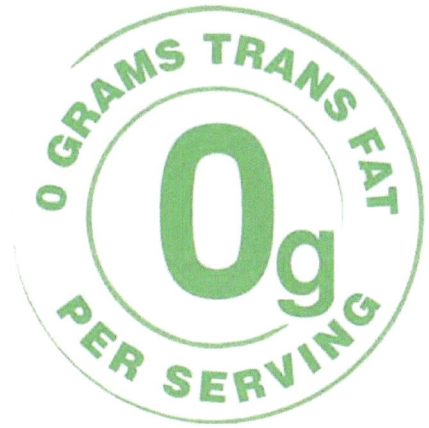

• Choose vegetable oils such as olive oil or canola oil
• Do not choose solid fats such as shortening
• Decrease the amount of fat used in cooking and at the table.

- Choose 2 to 3 servings of fish, shellfish, lean poultry, other lean meats, beans or nuts daily.
  . • Trim fat from meat and take the skin off of poultry.
- Choose dry beans, peas or lentils often.

- Limit intake of high-fat processed meats such as bacon, sausage, bologna & other cold cuts.
- Try the lower fat varieties.
- Limit intake of liver and other organ meats.

- Choose fat-free or low-fat milk and yogurt and low-fat cheese most often.
- Switch from whole to Non Fat or fat-free or low-fat milk. This will decrease the saturated fat   and calories but keeps all other nutrients the same.

- Check the Nutrition Facts Panel to see how much saturated fat, trans fat and cholesterol are in a serving of food.

- Choose foods lower in saturated fat, trans fat and cholesterol.
- When eating out, limit your intake of foods with creamy sauces
- When eating out, choose not to have dessert.

Keep in mind that with all of the fat-free products on the market today, that fat is still an essential nutrient.   The key again is to choose the right type of fat and to eat fat in moderation.   It is also important to remember that just because foods are fat-free DOES NOT mean they are calorie free or salt free. Salt should always be at the lowest or none.

A Little More Info on Sugar:

Sugars are simple carbohydrates and are used by the body as a source of energy. Dietary carbohydrates also include complex carbohydrates which include starch and fiber.

During the digestion process, all carbohydrates break down into sugar in the body. Some sugars occur naturally in foods such as milk (as lactose) and fruits (as fructose). Other foods have added sugars or sugar that is added in processing or preparation.

The body cannot tell the difference between naturally occurring sugar and added sugar but most foods containing added sugars provide calories and little in the way of essential nutrients such as vitamins, minerals and/or fiber.

Food containing added sugar can also promote tooth decay. Major sources of added sugar in the United States include soft drinks, cakes, cookies, pies and drinks such as fruit punch and lemonade, dairy desserts such as ice cream and candy.

❖   Names for some added sugars that appear on Food Labels include:

Brown sugar   Invert sugar
Corn sweetener   Lactose
Corn syrup   Malt syrup
Dextrose   Maltose
Fructose   Molasses
Fruit juice concentrate Raw sugar
Glucose   Sucrose
High fructose corn syrup Syrup
Honey   Table sugar

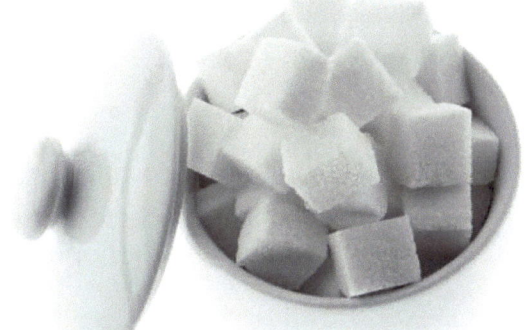

A food is likely to be high in sugar if any of the above names appears first or second in the ingredient list, or if several names are listed. Also available are foods with sugar substitutes such as saccharin aspartame, acesulfame potassium, and sucralose. These sweeteners are extremely low in calories. Remember through that some foods that contain sugar substitutes also contain calories.

Consuming excess calories from foods high in added sugars "may contribute to weight gain or lower consumption of more nutritious foods". The aim is to choose beverages and foods sensibly to moderate your intake of added sugar.

On Sodium:

Consuming less salt will reduce some people's risk for developing high blood pressure. Over 30 years of scientific evidence shows that a diet containing more salt per day is associated with elevated blood pressure.   Eating less salt can also contribute to a decrease in the loss of calcium from bone.

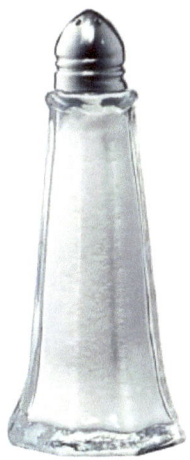

Sodium and salt are NOT the same thing.

Table salt is actually the common name for "sodium chloride". Table salt is 40 percent sodium and 60 percent chloride. Too much sodium can have negative impacts on health but on the other hand sodium has many essential functions in the body.

It include regulating fluids and blood pressure; transmitting nerve impulses and helping your muscles relax, including your heart muscle. The problem is that most people consume too much sodium. Only small amounts of salt occur naturally in foods. Most of the salt people consume comes from salt added during food processing: during preparation in a restaurant or at home and from adding table salt to foods before eating them.

A person's preference for a strong, salty taste is acquired and a learned behavior a very bad habit to brake. This learned behavior can decrease by gradually adding smaller amounts of salt or salty seasonings to food over a period of time.

The aim should be for a moderate sodium intake. Healthy adults need to consume only small amounts of salt to meet the sodium needs of the body. The Dietary Guidelines for is less then 2,300 milligrams per day. This recommendation is made to avoid excessive sodium intake rather to impose a restriction on the general population.

Ways to Decrease Salt Intake:

- Use herbs, spices and fruit juices to flavor food and cut the amount of salty seasonings by half.

- Choose fresh, plain, frozen or canned vegetables without added salt most often. Wash your canned food if possible to illuminate the salt.

- Choose fresh or frozen fish, shellfish, poultry and meat most often. They are lower in salt than most canned or processed forms.

- Always read the Nutrition Facts Label to compare the amount of sodium in processed foods. The amount in different types and brands often varies greatly.
- Look for labels that state, "low-sodium". They contain 140 milligrams or less of sodium per serving.

- If you salt foods in cooking or at the table, add only small amounts. Learn to enjoy the unsalted food.

- Consume plenty of fresh food.

- Drink water often. It is usually very low in sodium.

- When eating out, choose plain foods like grilled or roasted entrees, baked potatoes, and salad with oil and vinegar. Batter-fried foods tend to be high in salt, as do combination dishes as stews or pasta with sauce.

WATER

REQUIREMENT

- Eight 8oz glasses per day. Drink when your thirsty don't wait.

- You need more if you exercise, if you are overweight (drink 1 additional cup for every 25 pounds of excess weight).

- if you are sick or exposed to extreme hot or cold temperatures or if you eat a high fiber diet drink more water.

PROPERTIES:

- Water is the most essential nutrient the body requires to function.
- Every body cell tissue, and organ and every life sustaining body process needs water to function.
- Water makes up 60 percent of your total body weight and 70 percent of your muscles. Without adequate water intake, you cannot work at your top level of performance.

FUNCTION:

Water cools your body due to exercise, hot weather, etc.
- Water help to relieve constipation.
- Water is involved in all of the following: Waste transport, antibody transport, assists in food intake, blood pressure maintenance, nutrient transport, circulation of fluids, efficient digestion, hormone transport, lubricating body joints, electrolyte balance and all chemical reactions in the body.

WEIGHT LOSS:

- Don't wait until you are thirsty to drink water. Thirst means you are not drinking enough water.
- Use a straw to increase water intake as opposed to sipping from a cup.
- Take water breaks during the day instead of coffee breaks
- Drink water before, during and after exercise. Don't wait until you are thirsty.
- Carry bottled water around with you- when traveling, in the car, shopping, working.
- Not all water is created equal, read all labels on all bottled water
- Faucet water is the best water to drink. It still maintains all the minerals.

WATER FACTS:

Your body does not store water, if you consume more than you need your kidneys simply eliminate the excess.

- If your body does not get enough water that contains all the minerals you will experience dehydration which can lead to fatigue, muscle cramps, dizziness, headaches, and more serious consequences.

CALORIES

Calories are a unit of energy. The technical definition of a calorie is: 1 calorie is the amount of energy needed to raise the temperature of 1 gram of water by 1 degree Celsius.

A simpler definition is that a calorie is the amount of energy in food and the amount of energy the body uses. In food, calories come from only three nutrients: carbohydrates, proteins and fat. The calorie content of any food depends on how much carbohydrate, protein or fat it contains.

Energy sources	Calories per Gram	
Carbohydrate	4	cal/gram
Protein	4	cal/gram
Fat	9	cal/gram

PROTEIN

Protein like chicken, fish, meat, eggs, turkey supply amino acids. Amino acids help heal and repair our body. The more lean body mass one has the higher their metabolism or the faster they burn calories.

Protein also provides energy when carbohydrate and fat are in short supply. But if protein is being broken down and used for energy, it can't be used to maintain body tissue like lean body mass and the body metabolism decreases.

Adequate protein is important because it helps repair muscle tissue and all body tissues such as skin. To get adequate protein an individuals should consume protein at every serving and up to 6 servings a day to meet the requirement.

FIBER

Fiber is the structural and indigestible part of plants. Recommended fiber intake is 38 grams per day for men under 50 years old and 30 grams per day for men over 50 years old; 25 grams per day for women under 50 years old and 21 grams per day for women over 50 years old.

Unlike carbohydrates, fat and protein, fiber does not provide energy to the body and therefore does not contribute calories to the diet. Researchers have found that fiber-rich diets help protect against heart disease, colon cancer and diabetes and are beneficial in weight control.

There are two different types of fiber: water-soluble and water-insoluble.

Water-soluble fiber helps to delay stomach emptying, provides a feeling a fullness, improves control of blood sugar and lowers blood cholesterol levels. These include: nuts, legumes, barley and fruits.

Water-insoluble fiber normalizes intestinal transit time and increases fecal bulk. These include: bran, whole grains and vegetables.

The aim is to choose higher fiber breads, crackers, rice, pasta, etc. to increase daily fiber intake. When increasing fiber intake, gradually increase the amount consumed. Adding fiber too quickly or consuming too much on a regular basis may result in gas, diarrhea, cramps and bloating. It is also important to drink extra fluid when increasing fiber in the diet to help soften the fiber as it moves through the GI Tract and to help prevent discomforts.

Tips to Increase Fiber in the Diet:

- Eat a variety of foods. Eating a variety of foods ensures you consume a mix of both types of fibers.
- Use breakfast as a good time for fiber-rich foods such as bran cereal, other fiber-rich cereals, oatmeal, whole-bran muffin or whole-wheat waffles.
- Eat legumes or dried beans at least two to three times per week. Add them to soups, salads or casseroles.
- Eat at least five servings vegetables daily.
- When possible, eat the edible skin on fruits and vegetables such as on an apple or baked potato.
- Choose whole fruit more often than fruit juice.
- Eat vegetables raw more often or steam them only slightly. Over-cooking vegetables can destroy most of the fiber.
- Switch to whole-grain breads, cereals, buns, bagels, rice and pasta.

VITAMINS AND MINERALS

WHAT ARE VITAMINS AND MINERALS?

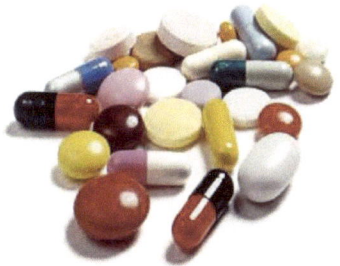

Vitamins and minerals are key nutrients to all the processes that take place in our bodies. They work together with other nutrients (carbohydrates, protein, fat and water) to make everything happen, including energy production, creation of protein and helping our body function normally. Unlike carbohydrates, proteins and fats; vitamins and minerals do not actually provide energy to the body but they are what help these nutrients provide the energy that they do.

Vitamins are essential nutrients that belong in two groups: water-soluble and fat-soluble.

Water-soluble vitamins dissolve in water. They are carried in the bloodstream and for the most part they are not stored in the body, at least not in significant amounts. The body uses what it need and excretes the excess through urine. Since the body does not store water-soluble vitamins regular intake can help to avoid deficiencies. Even though the body only uses what it needs and excretes the rest, moderation is still the best approach when taking supplements. Taking large doses of some water-soluble vitamins can still be harmful such as taking large doses of vitamin C from supplements, which can cause kidney stones and diarrhea.

Fat-soluble vitamins (Vitamin A, D, E and K- all others are water-soluble). They are carried into the bloodstream and through the body by being attached to fat. That is one reason it is important to have moderate amounts of fat in the diet. The body is able to store fat-soluble vitamins in body fat. For this reason, consuming too much fat-soluble vitamins can be harmful.

Minerals

Minerals are another essential nutrient that are needed to both regulate body processes and give the body structure. Minerals come in two categories: major minerals and trace minerals. All minerals are absorbed into your intestines and transported and stored in the body in different ways. Some pass directly into the bloodstream where they are transported to cells and excess is excreted in the urine. Others attach to proteins and become part of the body's structure such as in bones ad teeth. Because they are stored, excess amounts can be harmful.

WHAT ARE ANTIOXIDANTS?

As cells in the body burn energy they also burn oxygen and they form free radicals. Free radicals can damage body cells, tissues and DNA (our bodies master plan for reproducing cells), which could lead to the onset of chronic health problems.

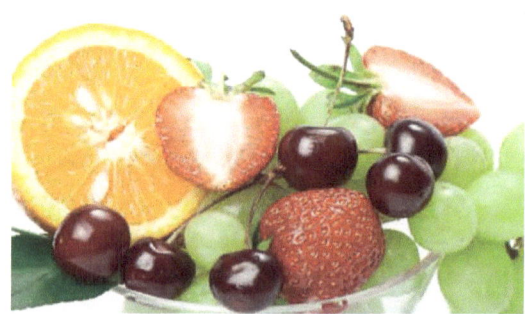

Certain environmental factors can also cause free radicals to form. Antioxidants are vitamins that counteract the effects of these harmful free radicals. Three antioxidant vitamins appear to play a important role:

22

- Beta carotene (the body converts beta carotene to Vitamin A).
- Vitamin C
- Vitamin E

Antioxidants seem to work together and complement each other.

HOW TO CHOOSE A DIETARY SUPPLEMENT:

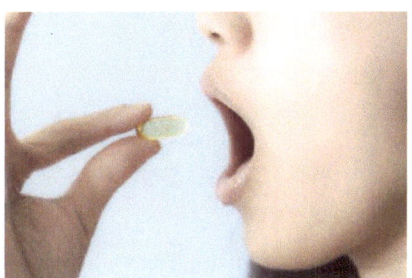

- Choose a vitamin-mineral combination.

Limit the potency to 100% or less of the RDA (Recommended Dietary Allowances). A supplement with 100% of the RDA is plenty, especially if you're eating a healthful diet or if it is less you may take is twice a day with food. Avoid large or mega doses.

- Choose a supplement the will suit your needs. Consider factors such as age, gender and medical status and activity level.

- Take supplements with meals to enhance absorption. When taking supplement always take after meals to enhance the absorption.

- Supplements do not work alone; they must have a carrier to take them into the blood.

- For economy, consider generic brands. Be wise and save money. Paying more for the same product generally offers no additional benefits.

- Check the expiration date. Over time, nutrient supplements lose some their potency.

- Take the supplement in the recommended dosage. Don't worry about missing a day of supplements, and never double up because you missed.

- Keep dietary supplements in a safe place – away from places where children may reach them. Supplements must be stored in a dry cold place away from heat and away from children.

- Supplements do not replace food. If you think that you can make up for a meal that you missed by taking extra supplements or replace a meal with supplements, you are dead wrong. Never replace a meal with any supplements.

- Food before pills. Always eat your meal prior to taking your supplements for optimum digestion.

- Advise your doctor about any dietary supplements you chose to take on your own.

Caution: If you are taking prescription medication, talk with your doctor before using dietary supplements. Supplements could interfere with the action of some types of medication.

CALCIUM SUPPLEMENTS:

- Avoid calcium supplements with dolomite or bone meal. They could contain small amounts of lead and other metals.
- Read the label to see how much calcium the product provides.
- Take calcium supplements as a supplement to ad to your meal or diet plan. Calcium Supplements can boost calcium intake, but they don't provide the nutrition needed to support bones.
- Nutrients your bones need: vitamin D, magnesium, phosphorus and boron.
- Milk provides Vitamin D, a nutrient that helps deposit calcium in your bones.

Take calcium and iron supplements at different times of the day. They will each be better absorbed when taken on their own.

- If you take more than one tablet, space them throughout the day to increase absorption.
- Drink plenty of fluids with calcium supplements to avoid constipation.
- Choose a powder capsule as oppose to a pill for better absorption.

Label Reading

1. About the Food Label

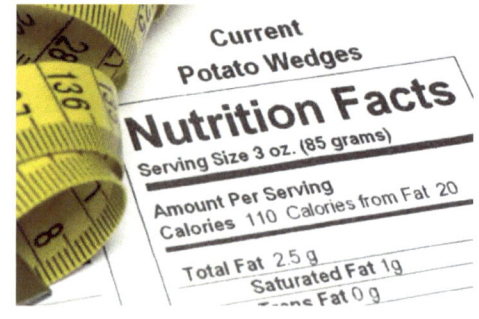

Under the Nutrition Labeling and Education Act of 1990 and regulations from the Food and Drug Administration and the U.S. Department of Agriculture, virtually all food labels must now give information about a food's nutritional content. The "Nutrition Facts" Panel provides information about nutrients people are most concerned about today. They allow consumers to choose healthier and more nutritious foods as well as to compare the nutrition of similar foods. The label enables people to choose foods for an overall diet that's varied, moderate and balanced. The food label is a great tool to help with weight management and good health.

2. Using the Food Label

Most of us are looking eating healthy and losing FAT / weight. Little do we know that there is help right at our fingertips. That help comes in the form of the Nutrition Facts Panel. The Panel is the rectangle box on a food label that provides consumers with detailed nutritional information on calories, macronutrients such as fat grams and calories, some micro - nutrients and other essential nutrients. It also offers the ingredient list, nutritional claims and health claims.

Note: NOT All of the information on the food label is regulated by the FDA and USDA to help consumers make healthier food choices for good health and a healthy weight.

You may use the Food Label to your advantage by following a few simple tips:

SIZE IT UP
The serving size and the servings per container.

▶ Ask:
   How many calories in a single serving? How many calories are in the container? How many servings do you plan to eat?

▶ ALL of the information on the Panel pertains to ONE single serving size.

▶ Eating two servings? Then you need to double ALL of the information including calories, nutrients and %DV (Daily Value). Your also doubling the fat and sodium too.

▶When comparing calories and nutrients on the same food but between brands, check to see if the serving size is the same.

Note: Many packages, including beverages, contain more than one serving. Each package is more than one serving. That can add up to a lot more calories and fat then you think, also keep in mind the sodium content.

%DV Footnote
FOCUS ON PROTEIN CONTENT

▶ Look at total calories and calorie from fat even on foods that you eat often and think you know well.

► Look at the total amount of PROTEIN in each serving.

► You may notice that when PROTEIN is high so are calories.

► When you look at calories consider how much of that food you truly expect to eat. If you will eat two servings ten you need to double all of the information on the label.

► Check to see how many total calories the food contains and how many of those calories come from PROTEIN, Sugar and fat.

► The fat source itself. Saturated and Trans Fats are the ones you want to limit while monounsaturated and polyunsaturated are healthy fats.

► Consider how PROTEIN per serving will fit into your overall intake for the day.
Note: The key is to keep your calories in check as you manage your weight. Keep in mind that if you eat and drink more calories then you burn you WILL gain weight.

► Calorie intake depends on your individual needs and the bottom line is how many total calories you eat by the end of the day.

► PROTEIN intake is always first and nothing but protein will help you lose fat and help elevate your metabolism.

However, in general, you can use this guide to gauge the calories in a single product
(based on a 2,000 calorie diet).

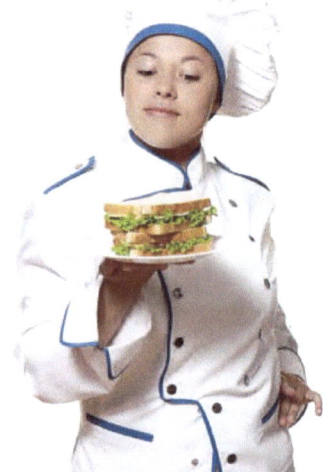

► If you choose a food that is high in fat and/or calories then balance your daily intake by choosing foods lower to calories and fat for the remainder of the day but always keep your protein intake high and sodium intake low.

MAKE YOUR CALORIES COUNT

When dealing with clients you want to make the most out of the calorie intake. Chose wisely and make sure the meals are always balanced. This entails choosing foods that will give you the most nutrition for your calories.

The Percent Daily Value (%DV) is a tool that can help you determine whether a food is high or low in a nutrient and ultimately if it is a smart food to choose.

To help you decide quickly use this guide:

5% DV or less is LOW
30% DV or more is HIGH

Get enough of these nutrients:

(The goal is to stay within 100%DV for each of these for every day)

Fiber, Vitamin A, Vitamin C, Iron Calcium, Potassium

Limit these nutrients:
(The goal is to stay below 100%DV for each of these for every day)

Total fat: Saturated fat, Trans Fat, Cholesterol, Sodium

*Note: Stick to mostly polyunsaturated and monounsaturated fats, healthy fats.

How do I calculate %DV?

Percent Daily value is calculated for you on every label. The %DV is based on the Daily Value or daily requirements for a 2,000 calorie diet. The Daily Values that are used to calculate the %DV are shown as a footnote at the bottom of each label.

For example if the label states 20% DV for sodium that means that one serving size of the food will provide you with 20% of the sodium you for the entire day or 470 mg. How much sodium you need daily is listed at the bottom of the label. The Percent Daily Value for sodium is 2,400 mg. So, 20% of 2,400 mg is 470 mg.

▶ Since the Daily Value are base on a 2,000 calorie diet, yours might be higher or lower depending on your calorie intake. The following is a chart of how the Percent Daily Values need to be adjusted according to calorie level.

Adjusted Percent Daily Values for Specific Calorie Levels	
Calories	Adjusted %DV
1.200	60 percent
1.400	70 percent
1.600	80 percent
2.000	100 percent
2.200	110 percent
2.500	125 percent
2.800	140 percent
3.200	160 percent

Note: There are a few nutrients that do not yet have a %DV. These include Trans fat, sugar, and protein.   But you can still compare total amounts between brands to pick the better product.

ASK IF THIS IS A SMART CHOICE?

Once you have checked out all parts of the label you need to ask yourself if this particular food is a smart choice.   Does it fit into a healthy diet and into your weight management plan?

- Is one serving size enough for me or do I need to double, triple, etc… the calories, fat and other nutrients on the label?
- Are the calories per serving low, medium or high? How many calories will be in the amount I actually eat and how many of those calories will be coming from "bad" fats?

- Are the nutrients that I need to limit low and are the nutrients I need more of high?

- Have I compared the label on this product to other Brands of the same to ensure I am getting the most bang for my buck?

- Should I look for an alternative?

The answer you get id different from person to person depending on the calorie intake, whether trying to loose, maintain or gain weight, and whether specific nutritional needs are concerned.

In your search for healthy products, have you often found yourself standing in the supermarket aisle trying to decipher a lot of confusion information?

Reading labels is very important to determine which items fit into your specific dietary plans. Consumer surveys show that most shoppers obtain almost all their information on food products from the labels themselves: therefore, misleading labeling can be detrimental to a healthy diet.

 For instant, a package of luncheon meat labeled 85% fat free may not be as healthful as you think. Fat content equals 15% by weight. Since fat is very light in weight, but very dense in calories, a slice of 85% fat free luncheon meat actually receives over 50% of the total calories from fat. If more than 30% of food's calories come from fat, it is considered a high fat diet. High fat intake has been linked to obesity, heart disease, diabetes mellitus and certain types of cancer.

Lowering fat intake is the key to healthy eating. In fact, research has even show that reducing fat intake to 10% or less of total calories consumed, can stop progression and even reverse arterial plaque build-up. So it's easy to see how important understanding deceptive labeling can be to determine which foods are really low-fat and which exceed your fat limit.

Terms such as lite, diet, reduced calories, no cholesterol, cholesterol free, are very misleading. Products labeled in this manner often offer only a slight reduction in calories or substitution of one type of fat for another.

The bottom line is that food labels enable you to compare foods based on key ingredients and there fore make healthier choices. Food labels allow you to include your favorite foods even if they are not always the smartest choices. If eaten in moderation and balanced by other smart choices throughout the day they can be included.

Use the Nutrition acts Panel to make your food choices easier and healthier!

Check this link out to learn more about the food label:

http://www.fda.gov/Food/LabelingNutrition/ConsumerInformation/ucm078889.htm

Nutrient label Claims

Nutrition label claims can help and explain and find foods that meet specific nutrition goals and help compare calories and other important ingredients.

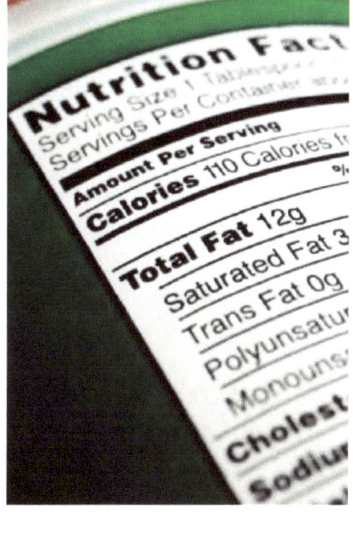

FREE: This means there is none or insignificant amounts of the following: fat, saturated fat, cholesterol, sodium, sugar and/or calories. This can also be worded as "without", "no", and "zero". If it uses "fat-free", "non-fat", or "zero fat" it must have less than half a gram of fat.

Light or Lite: On meat and poultry products, lite means at least 25% less fat. But on other products there is no standard meaning for Lite. It could also mean fewer calories, lighter color, less breading.

Natural: For meat and poultry products, natural signifies there are no artificial colors, flavors, preservatives or synthetic ingredients. On packages of baked goods, beverages and other processed foods, the term does not have to mean anything at all.

New: Meat and poultry products can call themselves NEW only for six months unless of course the manufacturer has not used up all of the company's New labels in that time. In that case they can be new for a year. Foods other than meat and poultry products can be new for as long as the product exists.

Salt-free: Only means no table salt added during processing, but the product could have significantly occurring levels of sodium or high levels from substances added for preservation or other purposes. Check the ingredient list for terms such as monosodium glutamate, sodium bicarbonate and Sodium saccharin.

LOW: A food can claim "low" in the nutrients if it doesn't exceed a certain level per serving.

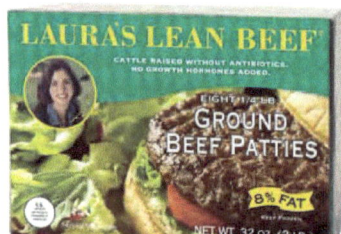

- Low-fat: 3 g or less per serving
- Low-saturated fat: 1 g or less per serving
- Low-sodium: 140 mg or less per serving
- Very low sodium: 35 mg or less per serving
- Low-cholesterol: 20 mg or less and 2 g or less of saturated fat per serving
- Low-calorie: 40 calories or less per serving

LEAN AND EXTRA LEAN: The terms are used to describe meat, fish, seafood and poultry. Try to choose foods in the lean and extra lean categories.

- **Lean:** less than 10 g fat, 4.5 g or less saturated fat, and less than 95 mg cholesterol per serving and per 100 g.

- **Extra lean:** less than 5 g fat, less than 2 g saturated fat and less than 95 mg cholesterol per serving and per 100 g.

HIGH: If a food has 20 percent or more of the Daily Value per serving for a specific nutrient, it is considered "high" in that nutrient.

GOOD SOURCE: If one serving of a good contains 10 to 19 percent of the percent Daily Value it is considered a "good source" of that nutrient.

REDUCED: For foods that are not naturally low in a specific nutrient, it can be labeled "reduced" if it has been altered to contain 25 percent less of that nutrient.

LESS or FEWER: This term can be used if in comparison this food is 25 percent less than the reference food for a specific nutrient or calories. For example, if chips claim 25 percent less fat or 25 percent fewer calories than other potato chips.

LIGHT: A food can claim this term if it has 1/3 fewer calories or half the fat then the regular product. Foods can claim to be light in sodium if the sodium content is reduced by at least 50 percent.

MORE: This means that a food has a nutrient that is at least 10 percent of the Daily Value more then the regular product or reference food.

HEALTHY: A food can be called "healthy" if it is low in fat, saturated fat, cholesterol and sodium. For single food items they must provide at least 10 percent or more of the Daily Value of vitamins A or C, iron, calcium, protein, or fiber. For frozen entrees and dinners, they must also provide 10 percent of two or three of the listed vitamins, minerals, protein or fiber in addition to being low in fat, saturated fat, cholesterol and sodium. The sodium content must be below 360 mg per serving for individual foods and 480 mg per serving for meal-type products.

Supporting clients goal

Nutrition affects general health status as well as physical performance, emotional feelings, as well as the actions behind all the mental behavior. There are strong links between all these activities that goes on simultaneously in the body.

Sound nutrition and its relationship with the body is very valuable and by being a personal trainer and a nutrition expert by providing safe and appropriate advice, you can change the lives and the emotions of every human being you come in contact with.

There should be no conflict between eating for health and eating for exercise. But each person is unique and each person requires a different approach. Prior experience and professional role boundaries must apply to the principles of nutrition in the context of safe professional practice.

Collecting information from a client is our first goal. We must analyze this information to be able to apply what is needed to each clients and their unique goal and symptoms.

First step:

A form must be presented to all clients prior to any analyzes or advice to proceed with what is demanded, and to understand the clients needs at the time for a better approach and a successful journey for a better health for life. Remember as you are the person they chose for help.

- All clients must sign a liability release form prior to any consultation
- All clients must provide a physician name to refer to for contact about their health.

Collecting information:
- Must always be confidential no matter what.
- Must be honest and complete or the program will not work.
- Monitored and collected every 2 weeks or every month.

Information collected:
- Obtaining consent from client
- Obtaining doctors info
- Obtain doctors release to exercise and plan nutrition
- Name and address
- Age
- Sex
- Height
- Weight
- Meals
- Supplements use
- Prescription drugs
- Allergies
- Meal replacement
- Body fat % (body fat measuring unit)
- Circumference measurement of body parts
- Rest time
- Sleep time
- Hours sleeping every night
- Personal goal
- Lifestyle
- Medical history
- Physical activity history
- Diet and meals history
- Food preference
- Nutrition knowledge, attitude and motivation
- Readiness to start
- Identify barriers
- Identify achievable goals
- Agree on goals
- Agree on help from others if needed
- Is this for emotional or physical gratification?

Liability Release form:

- All clients must sign a liability release form prior to any consultation
- All clients must provide a physician name to refer to for contact about their health.

Collecting information:

- Must always be confidential no matter what.
- Must be honest and complete or the program will not work.
- Monitored and collected every month.

What is a nutrition analysis?

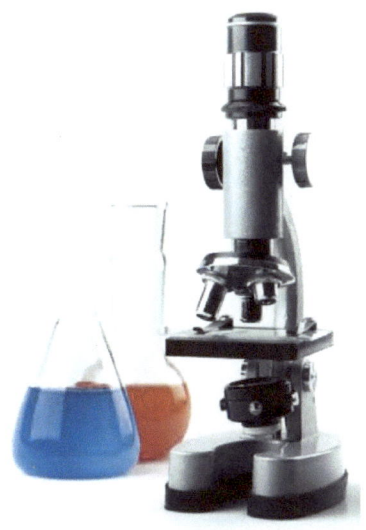

Nutrition Analysis refers to the process of determining the nutritional content of food. The FDA requires food manufacturers to display nutrition information on retail food products with Nutrition Fact Panel Labels, and soon the National Menu Labeling Law will require restaurants to display nutrition information for their menu items.

In the world of nutrition analysis there are two ways to calculate the nutritional content of a food sample; chemically, and by calculation. Chemical analysis must be performed in a lab where food is incinerated and tested for its exact nutrient content. Analysis via calculation involves taking data from ingredients that have been previously chemically tested and scaling those ingredients to match the amounts used in the final food product or recipe.

For clients that you plan to help with their daily food intake to help reach a healthy life style, nutrition analysis is about finding the proper food to the lifestyle they chose to have. Proper food to each individual is different. The amount of calories, protein, carbohydrates and fat can differ according to activity level or work accomplished during each day to how many hours of awake compared to the climate they live in.

To someone who is new to the analysis process, the details needed for generating nutrition information may be a bit of a shock. As someone who has been doing this for some many years, I have found the following things useful.

- Analyze solution
- Data base in a book form or computer
- Familiarize yourself with portions
- Familiarize yourself with other foods than the one you eat
- Always read labels to help you remember numbers
- Finally analyze your own food as practice

Gathering Nutrition data

1.1 Document and File Nutritional Information in Medical Records

- Maintain medical records using appropriate formats

- Enter and retrieve data using a computer data terminal

- Use current nutritional assessment forms

1.2 Interview Patients/Clients/Caregivers for Diet History

- Recognize different types of clients

- Plan and ask appropriate questions of clients

- Gather client information from family member(s) if possible

- Identify significant information and problems (allergies or diseases)

- Recognize nonverbal responses/cues

- Record information systematically and carefully

- Recognize ethical and confidentiality principles

- Gather client information from other professionals (doctors or nurses)

1.3 Conduct Routine Nutrition Screening

- Recognize routine versus at-risk clients

- Identify appropriate data to be gathered

o Utilize appropriate data-gathering format/approach for specific client type(s)

- Complete forms with client in an efficient manner

- Gather client information from medical record (if possible from a doctor)

1.4 Utilize Nutrient Intake, such as Calories and Sodium

- Perform routine nutrient computations using food composition tables

- Be familiar with all normal laboratory values and research

1.5 Identify Nutrition Problems and Needs

- Identify clients needing intervention
- Verify information to ensure its accuracy
- Follow up problems to address documentation
- o Identify food customs and nutritional needs of various racial, cultural, and religious groups

1.6 Identify Nutrition Needs if client is active or athlete

- Identify type of activity
- Identify activity level
- Identify how often the activity is per week
- Identify length of activity
- Identify location of activity (outdoor or indoor)

Apply Nutrition Data

2.1 Implement Diet Plans or menus Using Appropriate Modifications

- Translate nutrition plan into meals/foods to be served
- Modify menus to suit fiber content, texture, or feeding needs
- Modify menus to control for calories, carbohydrates, proteins, fats, and minerals
- Modify menus to suit medical or other personal condition(s)
- Modify menus to suit various racial, cultural, and religious differences

2.2 Implement Physician's Dietary Orders

- Recognize medical and nutrition terminology
- Demonstrate sensitivity to patient needs and food habits
- Provide needed diets from kitchen
- Determine availability of foods from kitchen
- Exhibit competency in suggesting the correct diet orders for clients
- Include patient input on diet prescribed by physician
- Recognize appropriateness of diet order for diagnosis

2.3 Apply Standard Nutrition Care Procedures

- Review client's nutrition needs, based on guidelines provided

- Verify nutrition content of foods

- Identify sources to consult to assist in implementing nutrition care plans

Provide Nutrition Education

3.1 Help Patients/Clients Choose Foods From Selective Menus

- Verify dietary requirements of patient/client

- Determine client's present knowledge and needs

- Choose appropriate resource materials

- Determine client's food preferences

- Suggest acceptable food substitutes

- Verify substitutes in terms of availability and facility practices

- Match food items identified with patient preferences

3.2 Select and Use Nutrition Education Materials

- Develop a plan for nutrition education (take time to sit and educate)

- Identify educational materials and resources (create and develop handouts for education)

- Use resource materials and equipment in teaching (books, pictures, videos, YouTube, websites)

3.3 Adapt Teaching to Client Educational Needs

- Verify client readiness and ability to learn (make it simple and easy, be patient)

- Ascertain background and knowledge of clients (clients may not be as educated as you are)

- Implement a teaching plan (educate on a continuous basis every week or so)

- Identify appropriate/available educational and social resources (library, internet, reports, email)

- Be open to communicating with clients at anytime (dinner, lunch, shopping …)

- Take your client shopping to help them chose properly the food that is needed

Food safety procedure

- Identify danger with storing food

- Identify danger with preparing food

- Identify mixing food

- Identify cooking temperature of food

Even though exercise and nutrition is your main focus, there are certain ways that nutrition can be discussed. Here are some tips to help you handle the topic with your clients:

Be a proxy. It is perfectly acceptable to relay national guidelines and dietary regulations to your clients.

Organizations you can seek information from include:

- MyPyramid.gov

- Food and Drug Administration

- Food and Nutrition Information Center

- Healthy People 2010

- Nutrition.gov

- National Cancer Institute

- National Diabetes Education Program

- National Heart, Lung and Blood Institute

- National Library of Medicine — Medline

- National Library of Medicine — PubMed

- USDA Center for Nutrition Policy and Promotion

- Weight Control Information Network

Know when to refer. When you find yourself in a sticky situation, it's time to seek counsel from an RD to protect yourself. Remember safety is your maid concern no matter what.

Sticky Situations

In some situations, it is best for a fitness professional to document a client's progress, then refer the client to an RD. Cases that involve eating disorders, morbid obesity, vitamin/mineral deficiencies, and food allergies can be best dealt with by a dietitian. It is often the role of a fitness professional to observe the warning signs of these conditions, helping to provide solutions to the disorder in its earliest stages.

- Anorexia nervosa can be identified by abnormal weight loss, excessive exercise despite weakness and fatigue, and a heightened sensitivity to cold temperatures

- Bulimia nervosa can be identified by depressive moods and altered eating patterns, especially binging on high-calorie foods. Unlike individuals suffering from anorexia, most bulimia sufferers are of moderate weight

- Trainers can observe other disorders, such as vitamin and mineral deficiencies. Although it can be difficult to identify a vitamin and mineral deficiency, symptoms such as muscle weakness, nausea, slow wound healing, and some skin diseases are considered indicators

Fees and charges for consultation:

As a business owner, you must charge for your services. Always collect for any services prior to scheduling an appointment. Sign up for a merchant account like Paypal, or other to be able to charge clients' credit cards.

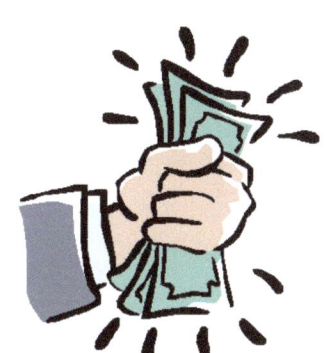

Dear Client:

Please read over this list of plans and choose the plan that suites you. If you have any questions please feel free to call me at any time to discuss.

Plan 1:   1 session = $ 250.00
        Includes one nutrition consultation and Body Fat testing.
        Paid at the time of service.

Plan 2:   3 sessions = $ 675.00
        1 session = $225.00
        Includes 3 nutrition consultation, and Body Fat testing.
        Appointments are scheduled in advance every 4 weeks.
        Paid in advance.

Plan 3:   12 sessions = $ 2400.00
        1 session = $200.00
        Includes 12 nutrition consultations, plus an eating menu plan and Body Fat testing.
        Paid monthly in advance beginning the 1st scheduled session over a period of 6 months   (session scheduled every two weeks).

Your Fee is always paid prior to scheduling and in advance.

If you miss a session, you will have the Saturday of the same week to ***make it up   between 12:00 P.M. And 4:00 P.M.*** depending on availability. I will also notify you of any openings during that same week to help you make up the session missed. Be sure that you keep your scheduled sessions because no other time slots are available. I am booked solid.

A 24 hour cancellation notice is required for cancellation of a scheduled session. Unless it is an emergency you will be charged for that session. But you will have the chance to make it up on that Saturday. Cancellation of a Saturday make up session will cause an extra charge for a full session to be added.

Thank you

RELEASE AND WAIVER OF LIABILITY / Example Form

Through individualized nutritional education and consultant support, my goal is to teach proper eating habits, good diet planning, daily exercise routines and a basic understanding of necessary nutritional requirements. I will also provide support and lifestyle change and management to successfully lose, stabilize and control weight / Fat. My nutrition program will teach people how to increase their metabolism, burn fat versus muscle tissue, eat healthier and do all this naturally

I will not recommend or support fad diets or diet pills, and I will constantly recommend support, participation and recommendations from our clients' **personal physicians**. It is highly recommended that you consult with your physician before beginning the program, and get a release form to start this program.

I, _____ , choose not to consult with a physician initiating my

relationship with this Nutrition and Weight management program and hereby release, discharge and covenant not to sue _____, its agents, employees, representatives, officers, directors, members and all other persons acting for their behalf, and all instructors, participants and advertisers [hereinafter called "release"] from all liability to me, my personal representatives, heirs, assigns and next of kin, for any and all loss or damage, and any claim or demands thereof on account of any injury to my person or property or my death, whether caused by the negligence of the releases or otherwise, resulting from my participation in the program. I acknowledge that my health and physical condition will allow me to perform the activities in this program.

IN WITNESS THEREOF, I have executed this release on the _____ day of _____ , 2011

SIGNATURE OF RELEASOR _____

Drivers License # _____

WITNESS _____

Nutrition History Form – Teen

Name_____

Date_____ Birth date_____

Address_____

City/State/ZIP_____

Phone Number_____ Email_____

School / Sports or Activities_____

Referred by_____

Reasons for referral_____

Health Care Plan_____

Primary Physician_____

Height_____

Weight_____

Body Fat %_____

Usual Body Weight:

Do you consider yourself:
1. At my goal weight/body composition for maintenance
2. At a weight lower than optimal for health and fitness
3. At a weight higher than optimal for health and fitness

Do you have a history of (check any that apply):
___Strict Dieting
___High Cholesterol
___Anemia
___Diabetes
___High Blood Pressure
___ Hypoglycemia
___Intestinal Problems
___Arthritis
___Asthma
___Food Allergies
___Lactose Intolerance
___Others (please describe):

Have you recently followed or do you currently follow any special diet? If so, please describe:

Please list any medications, nutritional supplement(s)/herbs, etc. you currently

take: Medication, supplement, or herb   Dosage

Frequency

- Please list restaurants where you frequently eat and how often you eat out:

- Who usually prepares food in your household?

- Where do you or someone in your house typically shop for groceries?

- Describe your current weekly activity/exercise routine:

ACTIVITY/PRACTICE   FREQUENCY   TIME

- List your Nutrition/Health/Performance Goals:

Please record two "typical" days of your food intake and activity on the sheets following.

- Day one:
  - Meal one:
  - Meal Two:
  - Meal three:
  - Meal four:
  - Meal five:

- Day two:
  - Meal one:
  - Meal two:
  - Meal three:
  - Meal four:
  - Meal five

Daily Intake Sheet

Time of Day	Food or drink	Amount	Preparation

<u>Type of Exercise or Activity</u>   **<u>Amount of Time</u>**   **<u>Place</u>**

How I felt today: Comments

Nutrition History Form: New Clients

Name_____ Date_____ Birth date_____

Address_____

City/State/ZIP_____

Phone Number_____ Email_____

Place of work_____

Referred by_____

Reasons for referral_____

Health Care Plan_____

Primary Physician_____

Height_____ Weight_____ Body Fat % (if known) ____

Weight Range Last 3 years:_____ 10 years:____ Goal Wt. Range:_____

Do you consider yourself:
1. At my goal weight/body composition for maintenance
2. At a weight lower than optimal for health and fitness
3. At a weight higher than optimal for health and fitness
Do you have a history of (check any that apply):

_____Strict Dieting   ___Anemia
_____High Cholesterol   ___Diabetes
_____High Blood Pressure   ___Hypoglycemia
_____Intestinal   ___Food Allergies
Problems   ___Lactose Intolerance
_____Arthritis   ___Others (please describe):
_____Asthma

Have you recently followed or do you currently follow any special diet? If so, please describe:

Nutrition History Form: New Client, p. 2

Please list any medications, nutritional supplement(s)/herbs, etc. you currently take:

Medication, supplement, or herb   Dosage   Frequency

Please list restaurants where you frequently eat and how often you eat out:

Who usually prepares food in your household?

Where do you typically shop for groceries?

Describe your current weekly activity/exercise routine:

ACTIVITY	FREQUENCY	TIME

List your Nutrition/Health Goals:

Please record two "typical" days of your food intake and activity on the sheets following.

Daily Intake Sheet

Time of Day	Food or drink	Amount	Preparation

Type of Exercise or Activity   **Amount of Time**   **Place**

How I felt today:

Comments:

CLIENT REFERENCE

NAME_____CLIENT #_____

ADDRESS_____

CITY_____ZIP_____

PHONE_____BUS_____

CELL_____FAX_____

PAGER_____REFFERRED BY_____

EMPLOYER_____

AGE_____DATE OF BIRTH_____HT____'____"WEIGHT____LBS

WEEK	SERVICE	CHARGE	CHECK	CASH	BALANCE
1					
2					
3					
4					
5					
6					
7					
8					
9					
10					
11					
12					

Long Term Statistic and Fitness Information

NAME:_____ ***DATE:***_____

Counselor:_____

Trainer / Nutritionist:_____

Goal:

Body Fat:_____
Weight:_____

DATE						
BODY FAT						
WEIGHT						
NECK						
SHOULDER						
CHEST						
WAIST						
HIPS						
THIGHS						
CALVES						
BICEPS RELAXED						
BICEPS FLEXED						
PULSE RATE						
BLOOD PRESSURE						

Shopping List

If you are allergic to any of the foods listed below, please advise your consultant prior to starting on your program

Proteins: 4 meals a day

Skinless chicken, eggs, turkey, lean cut beef, albacore, cod, orange roughy, salmon, tuna, crab, shrimp, soy isolate protein powder, peanut butter.

Carbohydrates: 2 early day meal

Sweet potatoes, oatmeal, yams, apples, bananas, cantaloupe, grapefruit, oranges, watermelon, strawberries.

Vegetables (high fiber):

Alfalfa sprout, broccoli, cauliflower, cucumbers, eggplants, lettuce, mushrooms, celery, peppers, onions, radishes, spinach, zucchini, and tomatoes, avocado.

Beverages:

Only diet beverages are acceptable. Do not drink any alcohol until advised by your technician. Drink plenty of water, Ice tea and coffee, are encouraged.

This program will work only if you change your eating habits. Please give yourself at least one to two months to adjust from your habitual eating. The will to succeed is to apply the recommendations that are asked of you.

IMPORTANT:

DO NOT EAT ANY OF THE FOLLOWING AT ANY TIME:

Pasta, dairy products, salt, pancakes, bagels, breads, beans, ice creams, shakes, pastries, cookies, fried foods, soy sauce, catsup, fat free or lite mayonnaise, salad dressings.

Confidential Activity Records:

This page must always stay in your clients file at your office for recording all activities and discussions that you have between you and the client at anytime. Even phone calls must be recorded with time and date.

This is for your protection and must be done. Don't be lazy.

Insulin role in the human body. Insulin plays many roles.

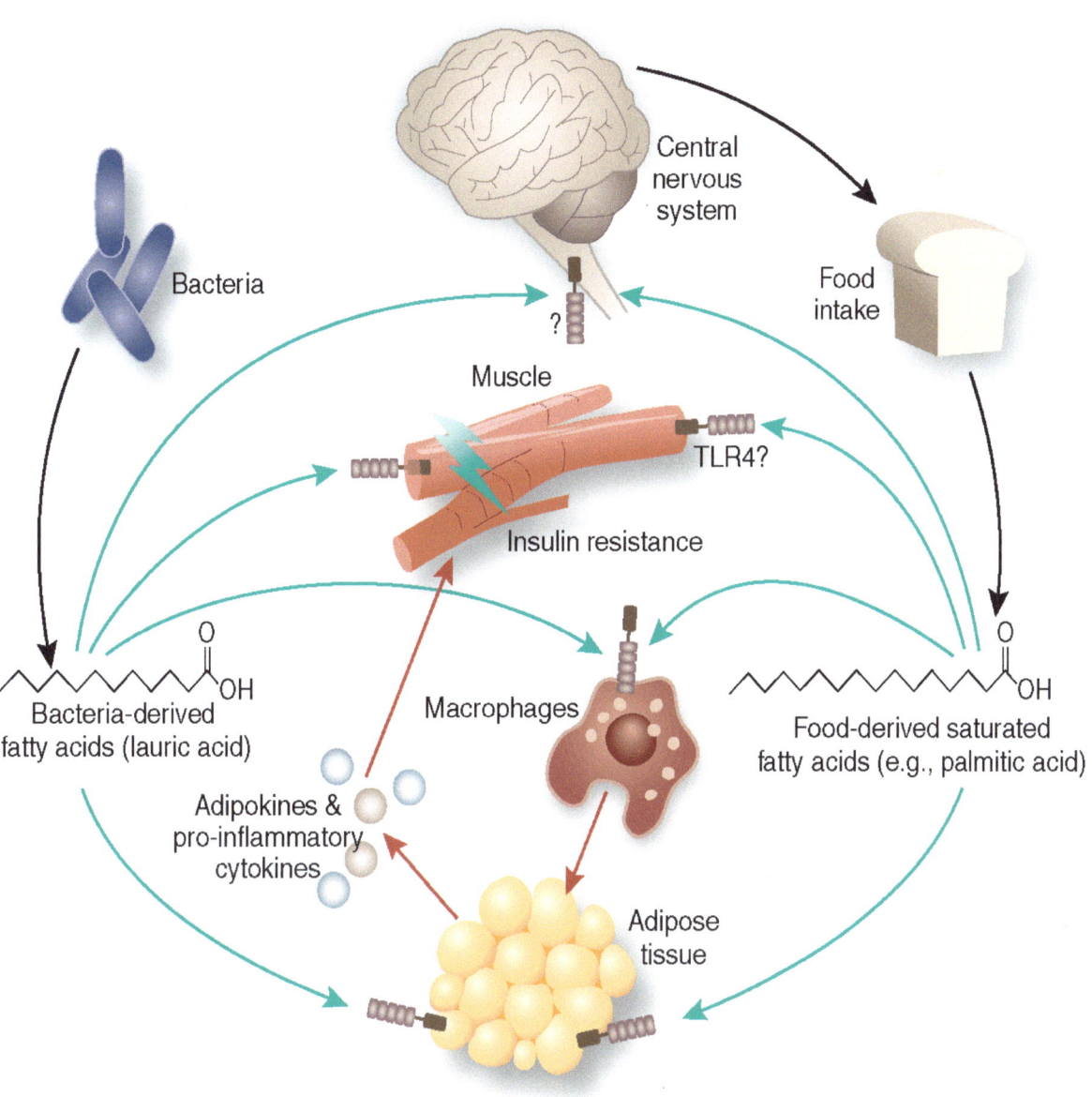

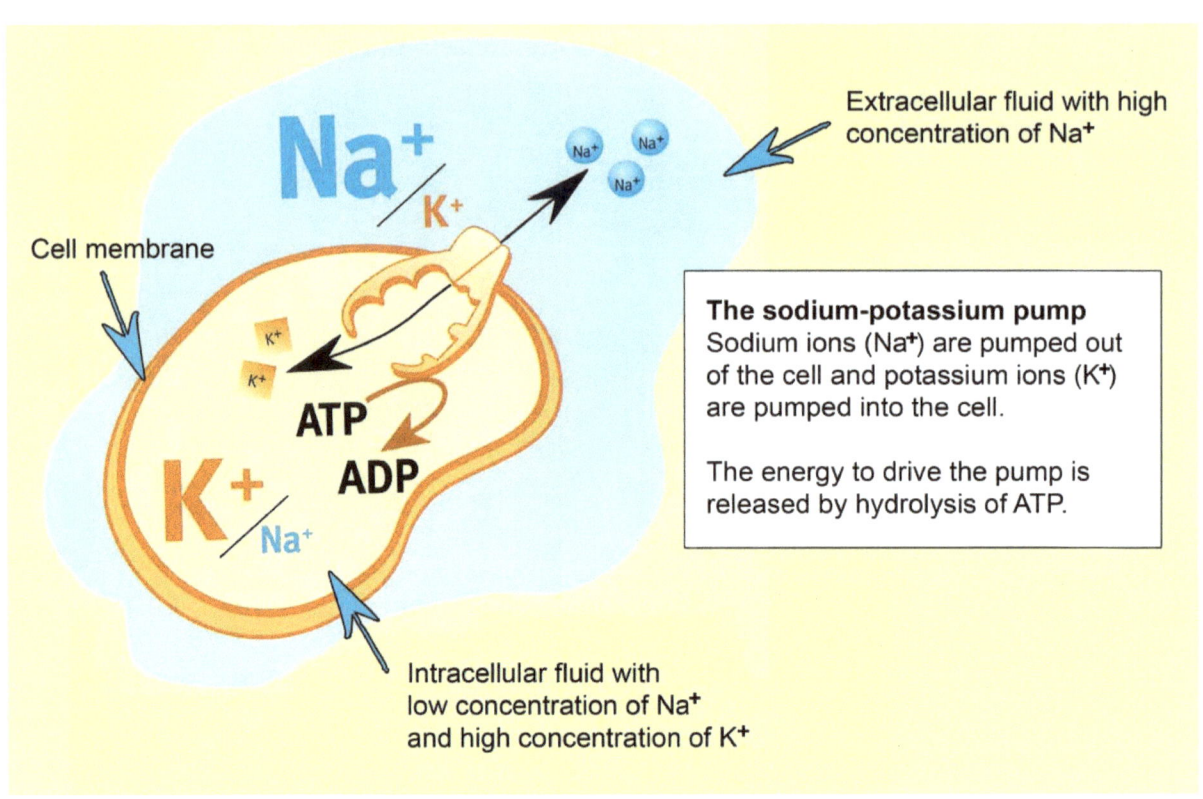

Extracellular fluid with high concentration of Na⁺

Cell membrane

The sodium-potassium pump
Sodium ions (Na⁺) are pumped out of the cell and potassium ions (K⁺) are pumped into the cell.

The energy to drive the pump is released by hydrolysis of ATP.

Intracellular fluid with low concentration of Na⁺ and high concentration of K⁺

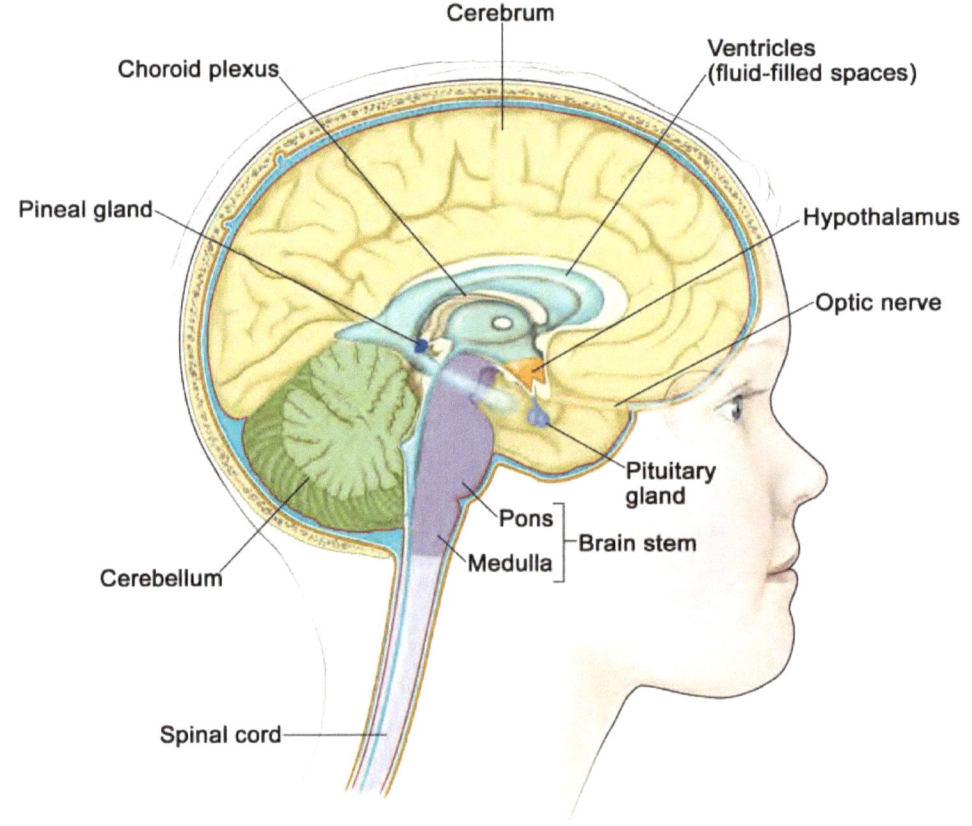

Cerebrum

Ventricles (fluid-filled spaces)

Choroid plexus

Pineal gland

Hypothalamus

Optic nerve

Pituitary gland

Pons

Medulla

Brain stem

Cerebellum

Spinal cord

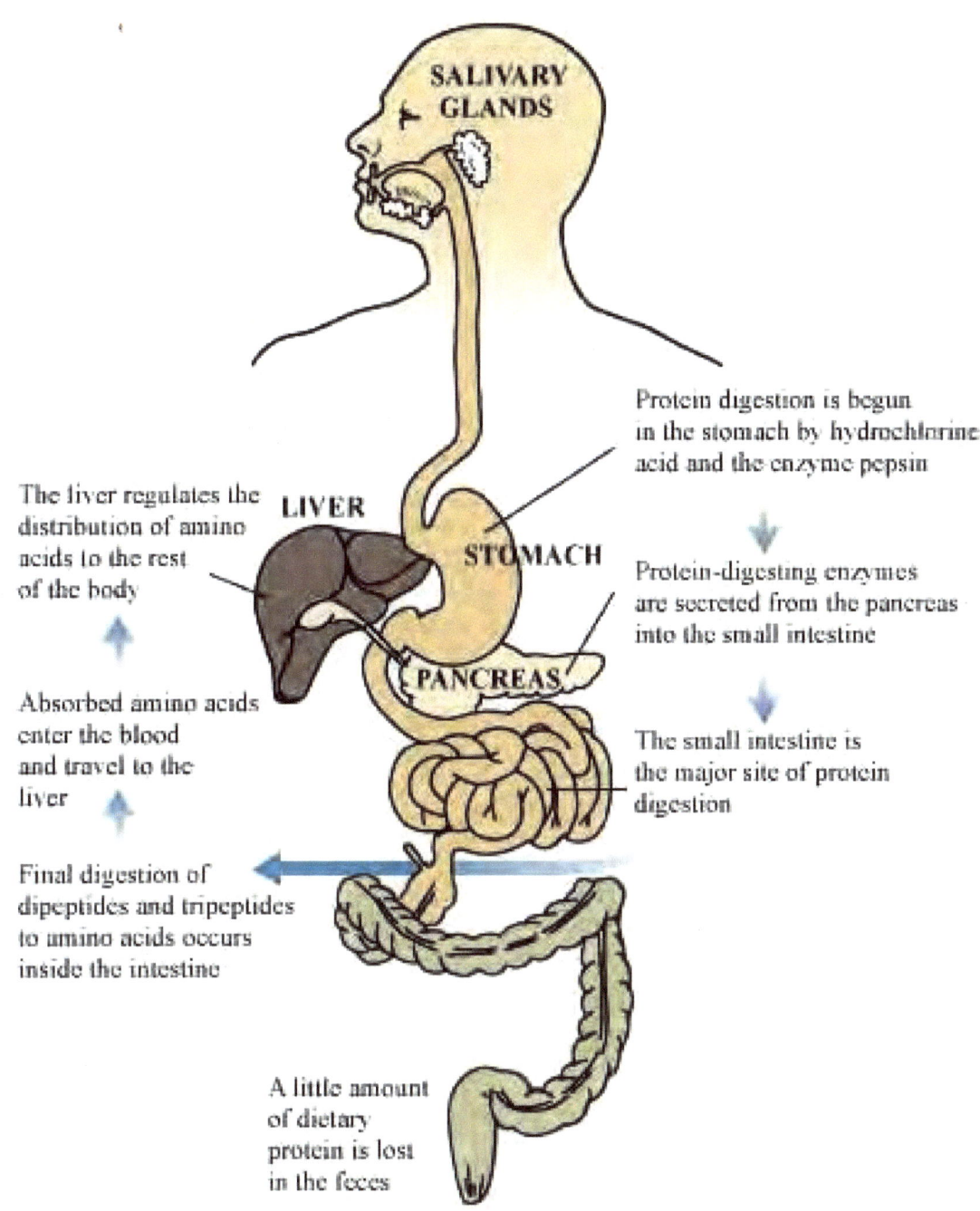

SALIVARY GLANDS

Protein digestion is begun in the stomach by hydrochlorine acid and the enzyme pepsin

The liver regulates the distribution of amino acids to the rest of the body

LIVER

STOMACH

Protein-digesting enzymes are secreted from the pancreas into the small intestine

Absorbed amino acids enter the blood and travel to the liver

PANCREAS

The small intestine is the major site of protein digestion

Final digestion of dipeptides and tripeptides to amino acids occurs inside the intestine

A little amount of dietary protein is lost in the feces

The Endocrine System

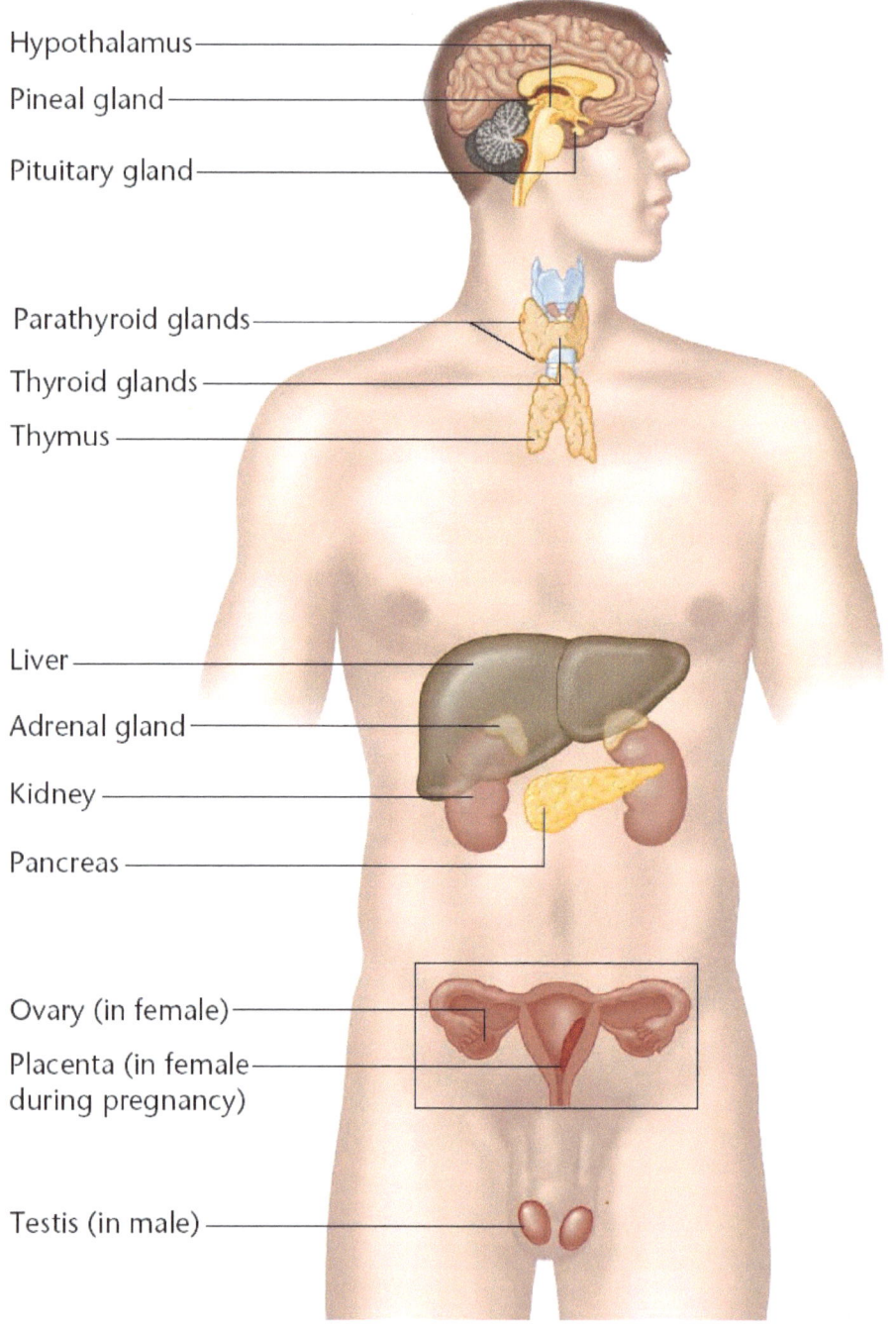

Hypothalamus

Pineal gland

Pituitary gland

Parathyroid glands

Thyroid glands

Thymus

Liver

Adrenal gland

Kidney

Pancreas

Ovary (in female)

Placenta (in female during pregnancy)

Testis (in male)

Protein Synthesis

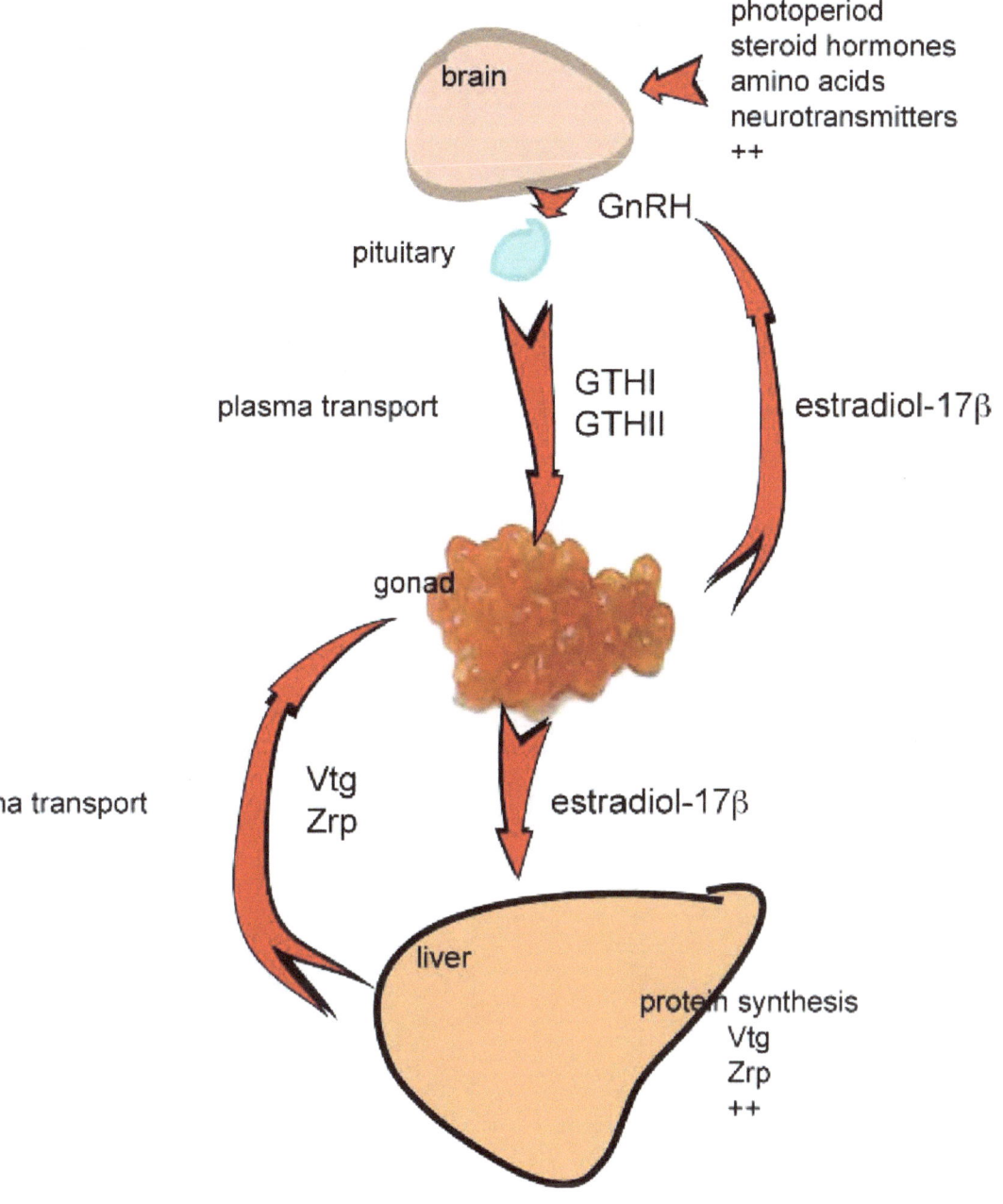

brain

photoperiod
steroid hormones
amino acids
neurotransmitters
++

GnRH

pituitary

plasma transport

GTHI
GTHII

estradiol-17β

gonad

Vtg
Zrp

plasma transport

estradiol-17β

liver

protein synthesis
Vtg
Zrp
++

Gastric Bypass

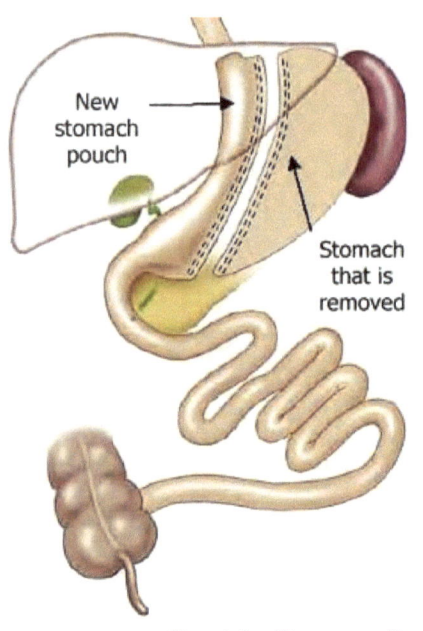

New stomach pouch

Stomach that is removed

Gastric Band Pump

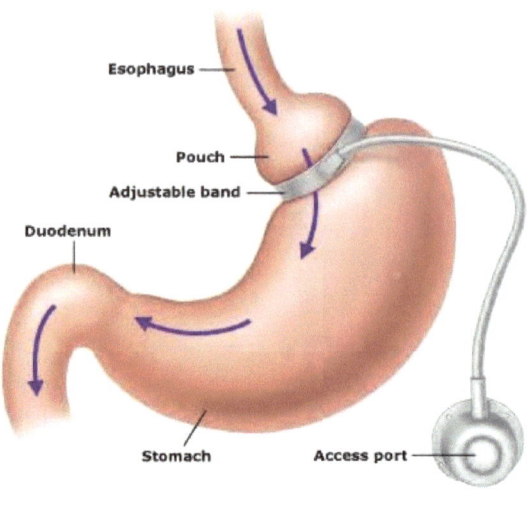

Esophagus

Pouch

Adjustable band

Duodenum

Stomach

Access port

Gastric Bypass Surgery

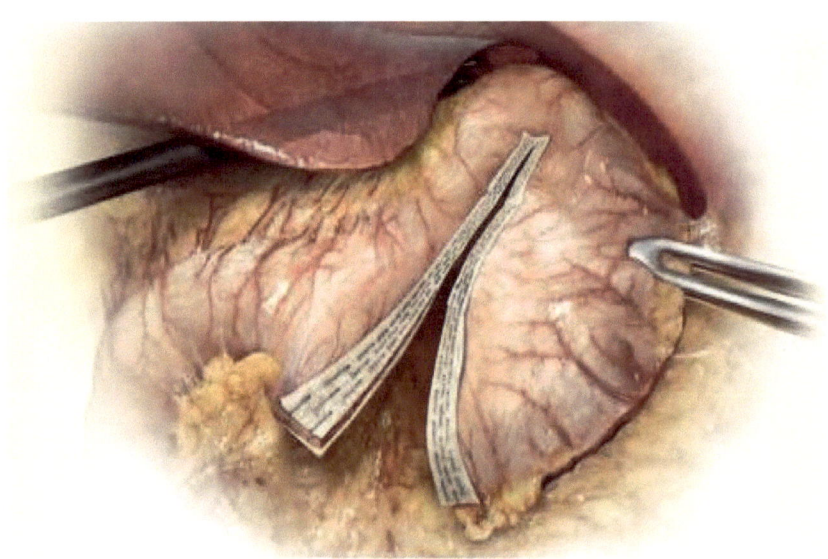

Pancreas – liver – Gall Bladder – Stomach

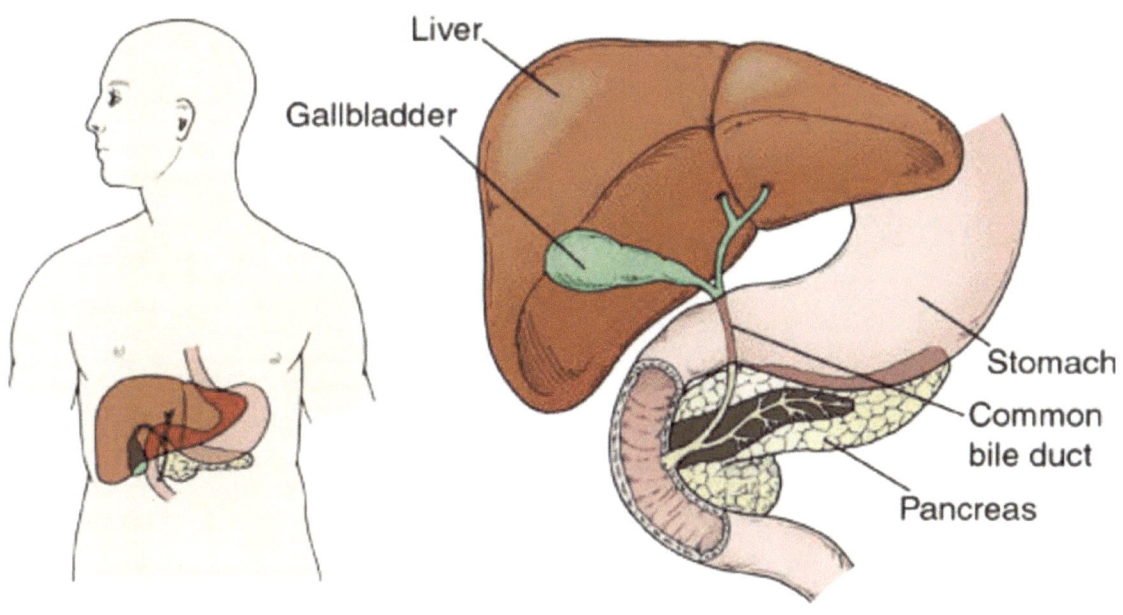

Liver
Gallbladder
Stomach
Common bile duct
Pancreas

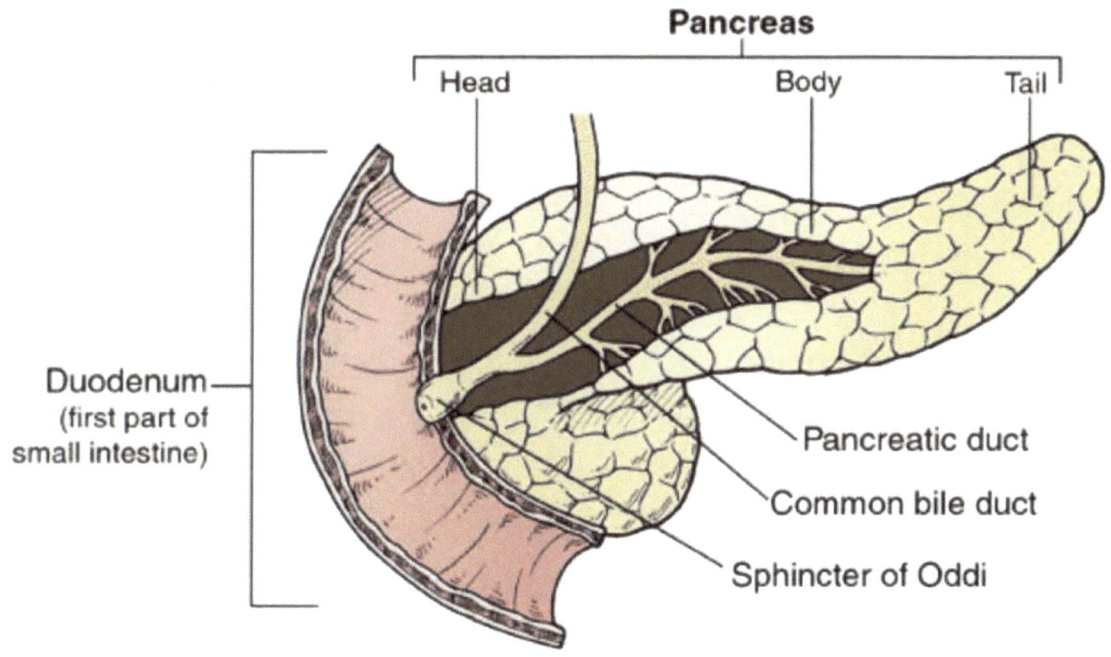

Pancreas

Head   Body   Tail

Duodenum
(first part of
small intestine)

Pancreatic duct
Common bile duct
Sphincter of Oddi

Anatomy of the Liver

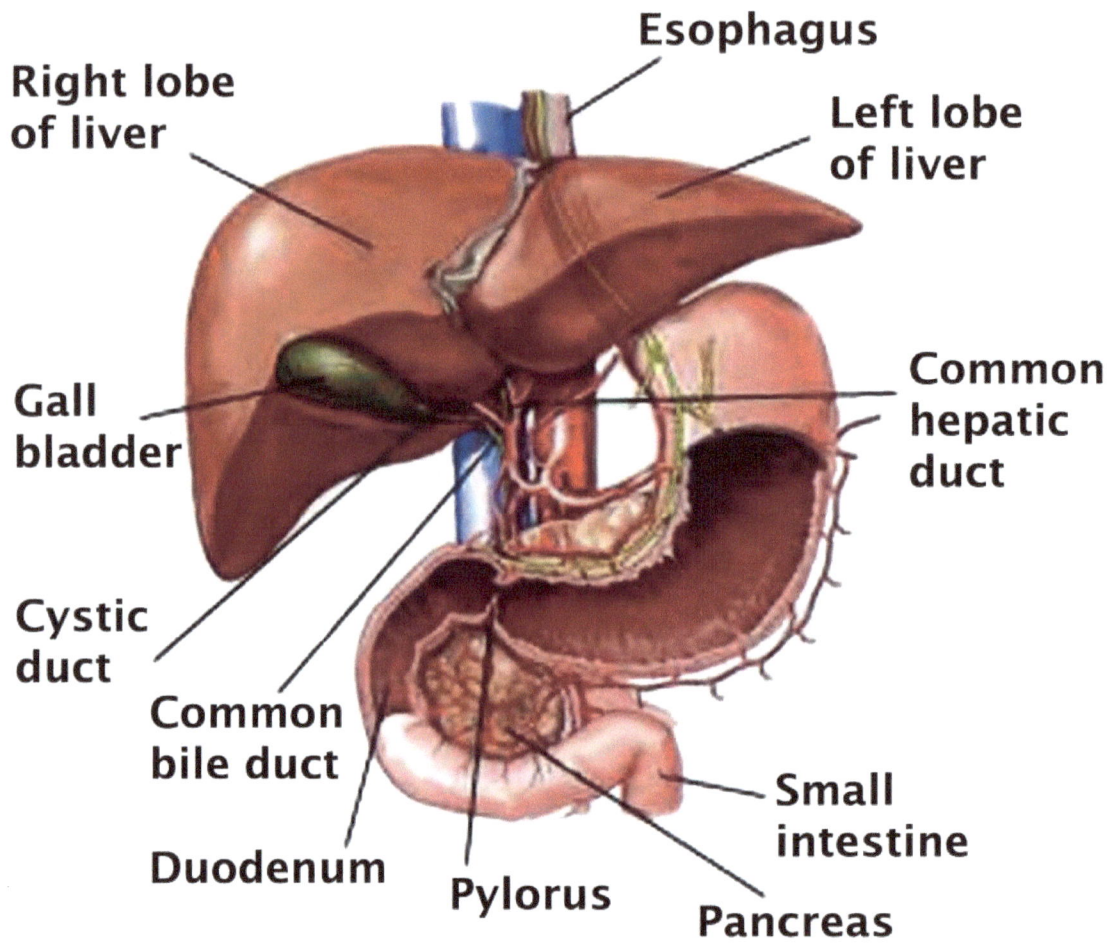

Esophagus

Right lobe
of liver

Left lobe
of liver

Common
hepatic
duct

Gall
bladder

Cystic
duct

Common
bile duct

Small
intestine

Duodenum

Pylorus

Pancreas

Cortisol Catabolism

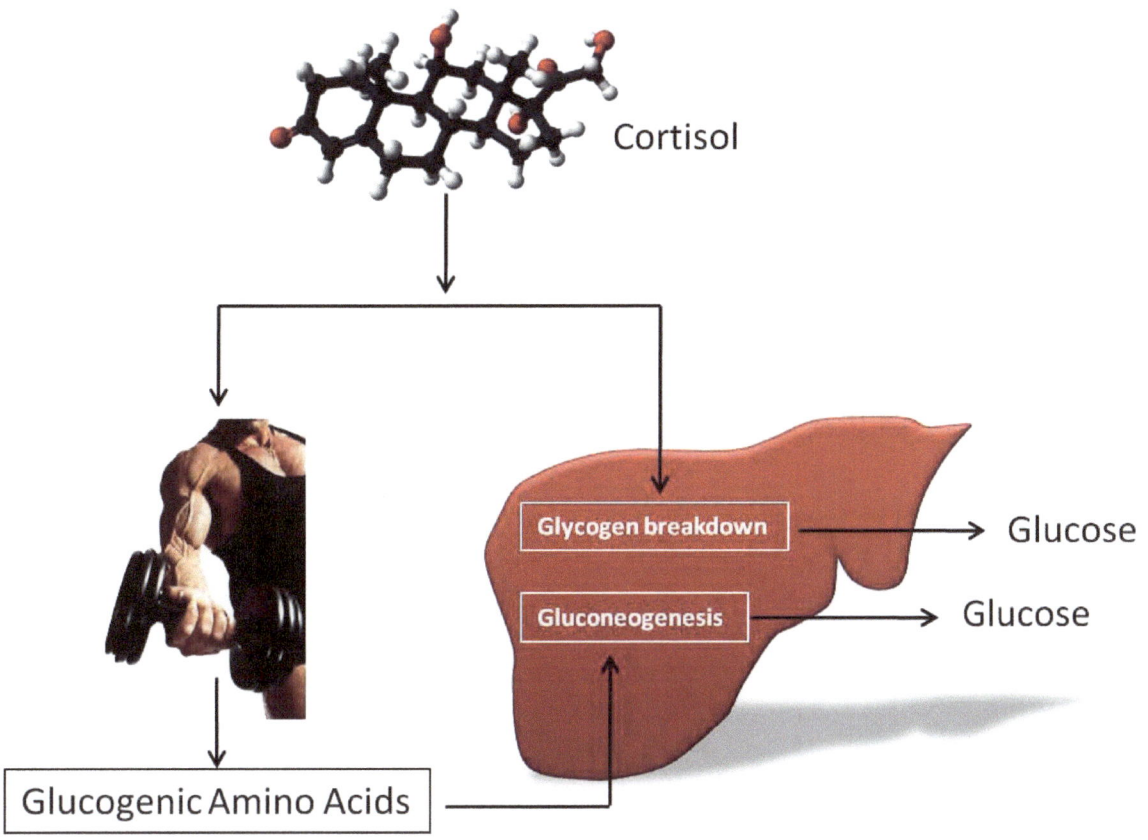

Cortisol

Glycogen breakdown → Glucose

Gluconeogenesis → Glucose

Glucogenic Amino Acids

The Personal Trainers Association
www.propta.com
www.personaltrainerscertification.com

info@propta.com

Office: 877-317-3577
Office: 818-766-3317

FAX: 877-533-7540